Traditional Chinese Medicine and Pharmacology

By FU WEIKANG

FOREIGN LANGUAGES PRESS BEIJING

First edition 1985

ISBN 0-8351-1351-5

Published by the Foreign Languages Press
24 Baiwanzhuang Road, Beijing, China

Printed by the Foreign Languages Printing House
19 West Chegongzhuang Road, Beijing, China

Distributed by the China International Book Trading Corporation
(Guoji Shudian), P.O. Box 399, Beijing, China

Printed in the People's Republic of China

CONTENTS

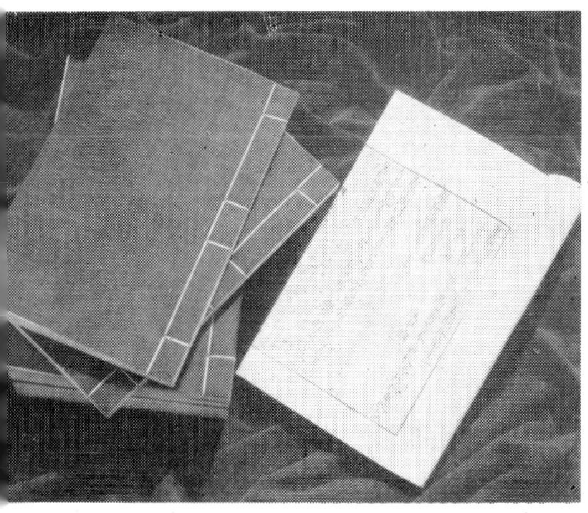

The Yellow Emperor's Canon of Medicine, the earliest medical book extant in China. This is a copy block-printed in the 16th century.

Passages in *The Yellow Emperor's Canon of Medicine* dealing with preventive medicine.

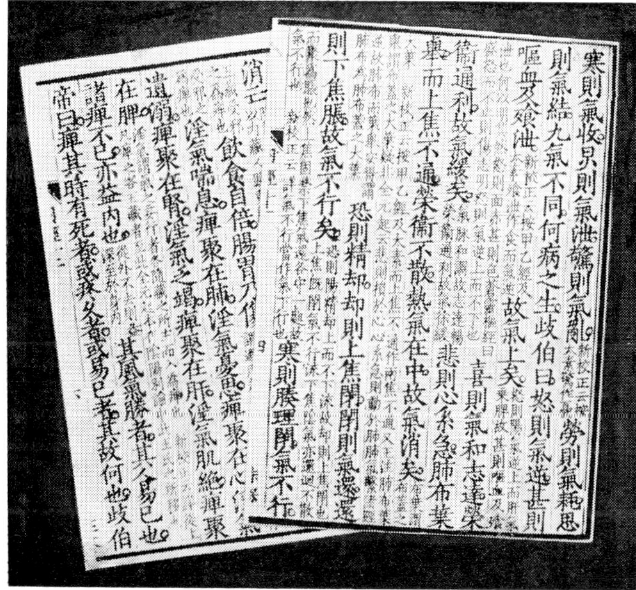

寒則氣收炅則氣泄驚則氣亂勞則氣耗思
則氣結九氣不同何病之生岐伯曰怒則氣逆甚則
嘔血及飧泄故氣上矣
喜則氣和志達榮
衛通利故氣緩矣
悲則心系急肺布葉
舉而上焦不通榮衛不散熱氣在中故氣消矣
恐則精卻卻則上焦閉閉則氣還還
則下焦脹故氣不行矣
寒則腠理閉氣不行

消
飲食自倍腸胃乃傷
淫氣喘息痹聚在肺淫氣憂思痹聚在心
遺溺痹聚在腎淫氣乏竭痹聚在肝淫氣肌絕痹聚
在脾
諸痹不已亦益內也
其風氣勝者其人易已也
帝曰痹其時有死者或疼久者或易已者其故何也岐伯

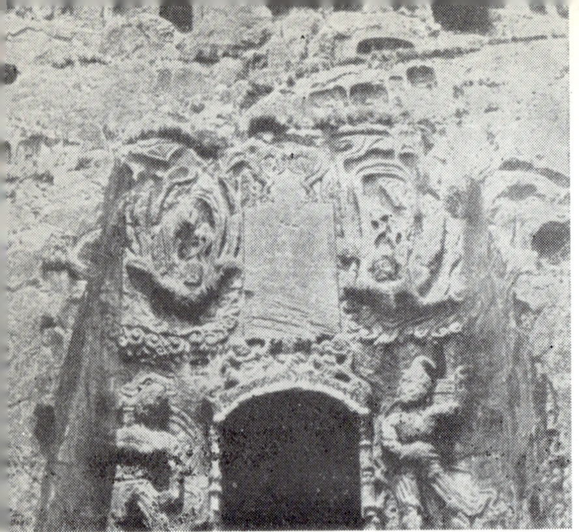

"The Cave of the Dragon Gate Prescriptions", at Luoyang, Henan Province, where prescriptions are engraved on stone.

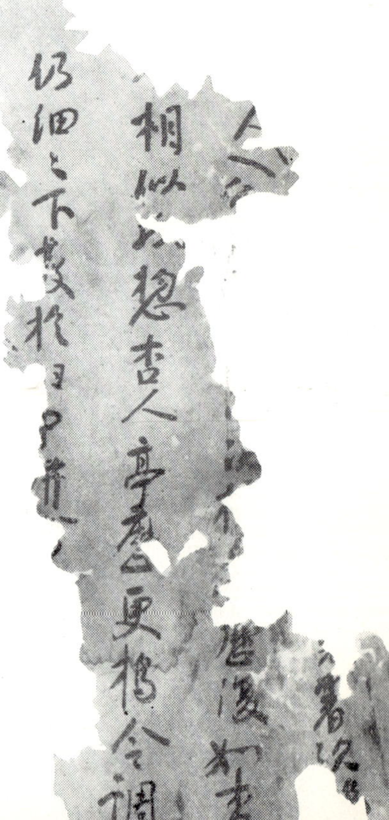

Fragments of a 1,000-year-old Chinese prescription of the Tang Dynasty unearthed in Turpan, Xinjiang.

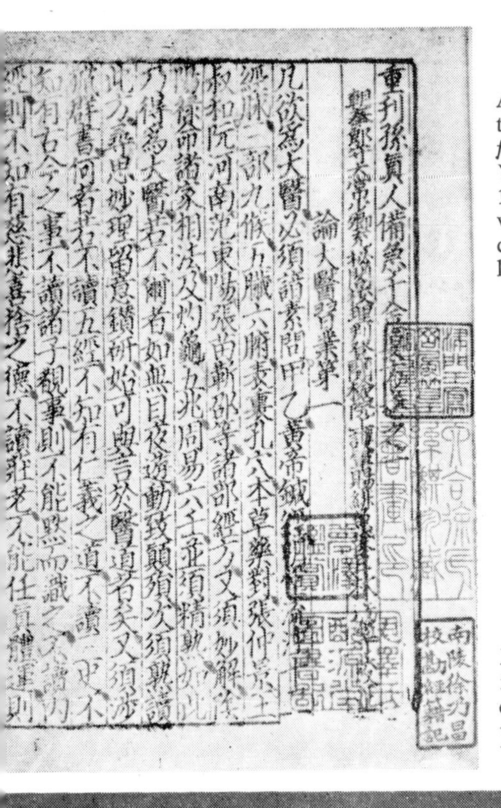

重刊孫眞人備急千金要方卷第一

朝奉郎守太常少卿充秘閣校理判登聞檢院上護軍賜緋魚袋臣林億等校正

論大醫習業第一

凡欲為大醫必須諳素問甲乙黃帝鍼經明堂流注十二經脈三部九候五藏六府表裏孔穴本草藥對張仲景王叔和阮河南范東陽張苗靳邵等諸部經方又須妙解陰陽祿命諸家相法及灼龜五兆周易六壬並須精熟如此乃得為大醫若不爾者如無目夜遊動致顛殞次須熟讀此方尋思妙理留意鑽研始可與言於醫道者矣又須涉獵群書何者若不讀五經不知有仁義之道不讀三史不知有古今之事不讀諸子睹事則不能默而識之不讀內經則不知有慈悲喜捨之德不讀莊老不能任眞體運則

A block-printed copy of the *Golden Prescriptions for Emergencies* of the Yuan Dynasty (1271-1368). The book was written by the famous doctor Sun Simiao who lived in the 7th century.

Boxes for keeping medicine discovered in a cellar of the Tang Dynasty (618-907). In the boxes is frankincense.

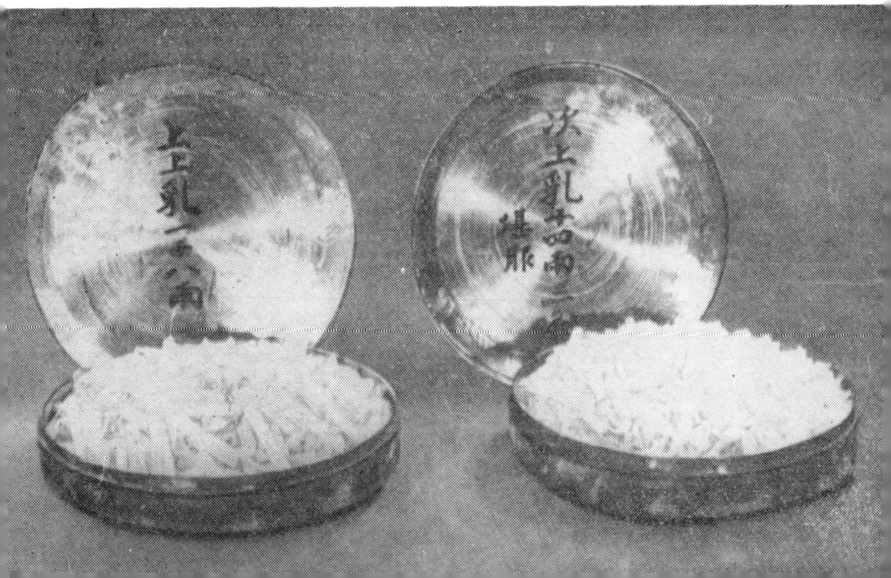

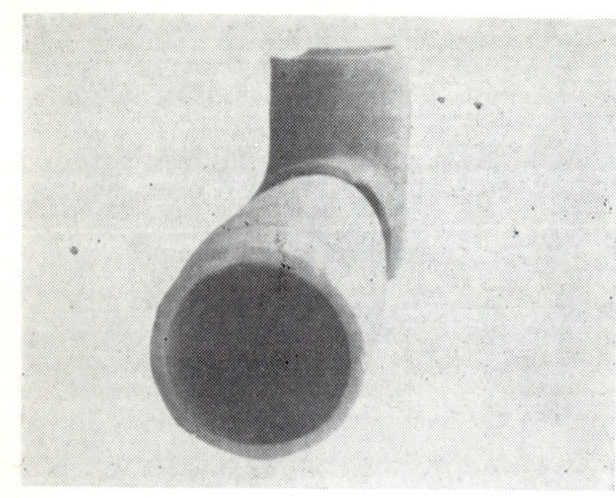

Sewage pipe of the Han Dynasty unearthed in Xianyang, Shaanxi Province, in 1958.

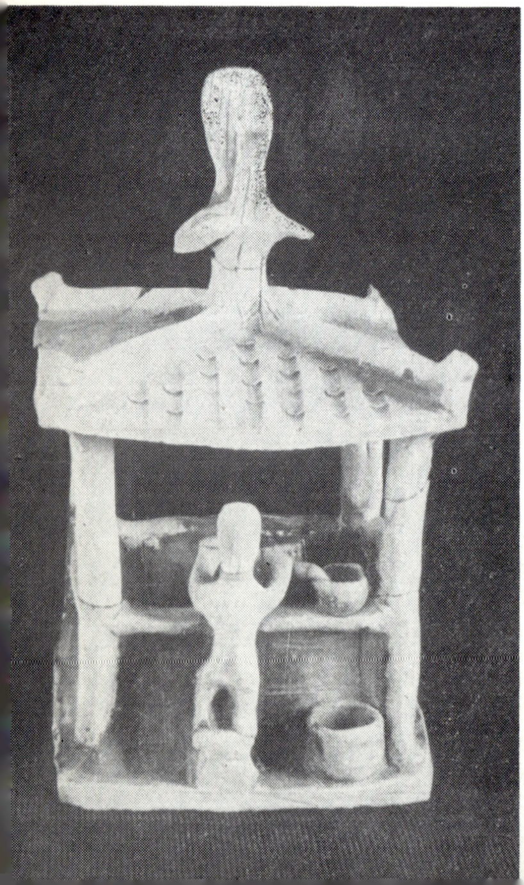

A model of a well made of pottery unearthed in a Han tomb (206 B.C.-A.D. 220).

Bottle gourds in which Chinese medicine was kept.

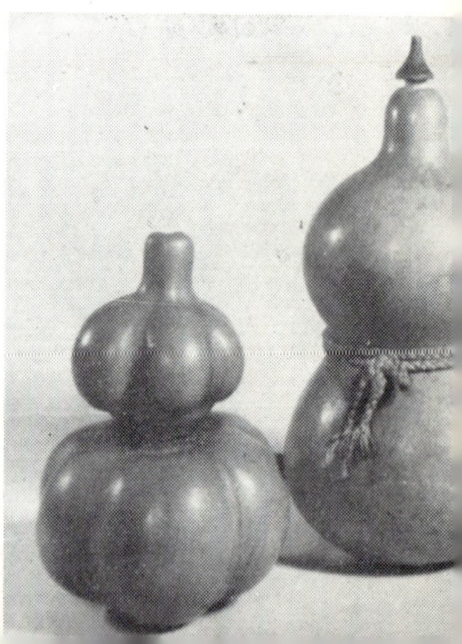

Indoor incense burner of the Ming Dynasty for fuming away disease factors.

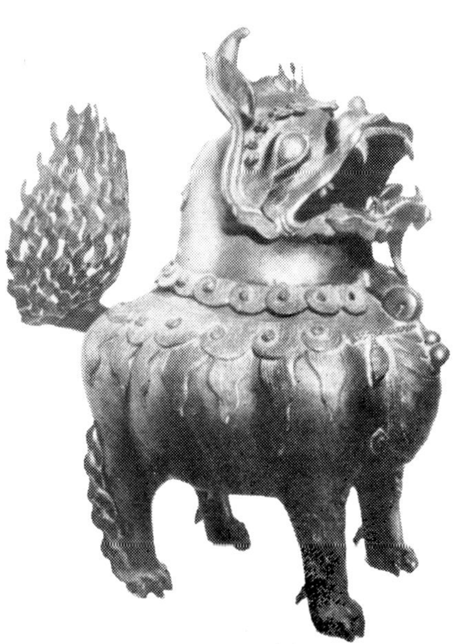

The front and back of a rattle used by roving doctors when they roamed the streets offering to give treatment.

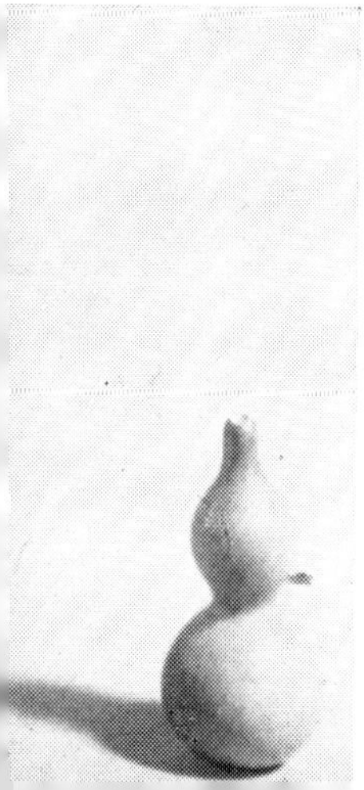

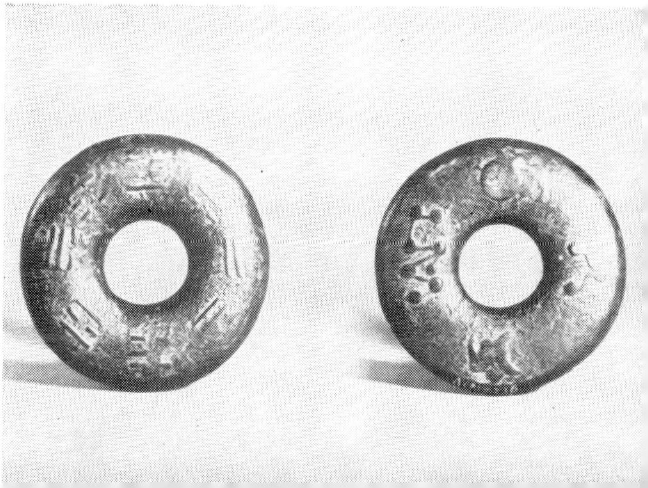

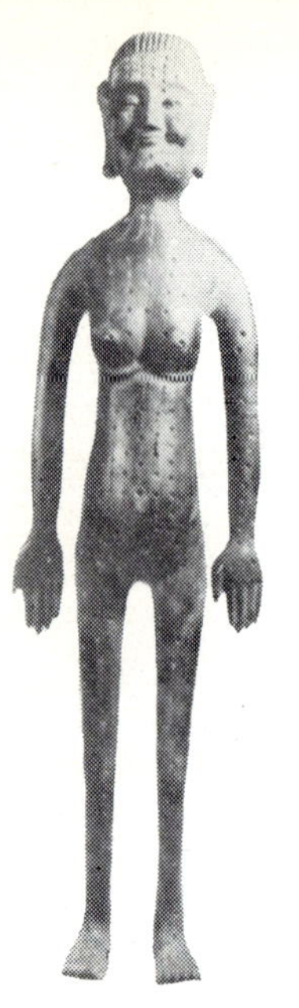

Bronze acupuncture manikin used as award by the Qing government in 1744.

Ancient Chinese surgical instruments.

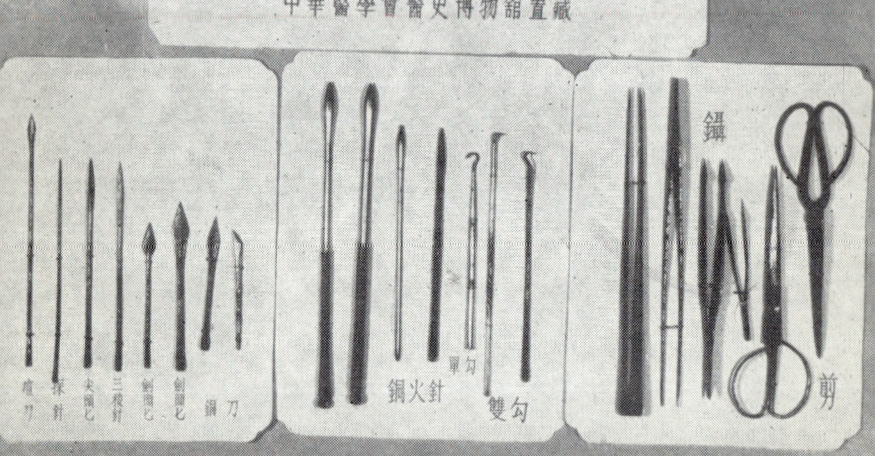

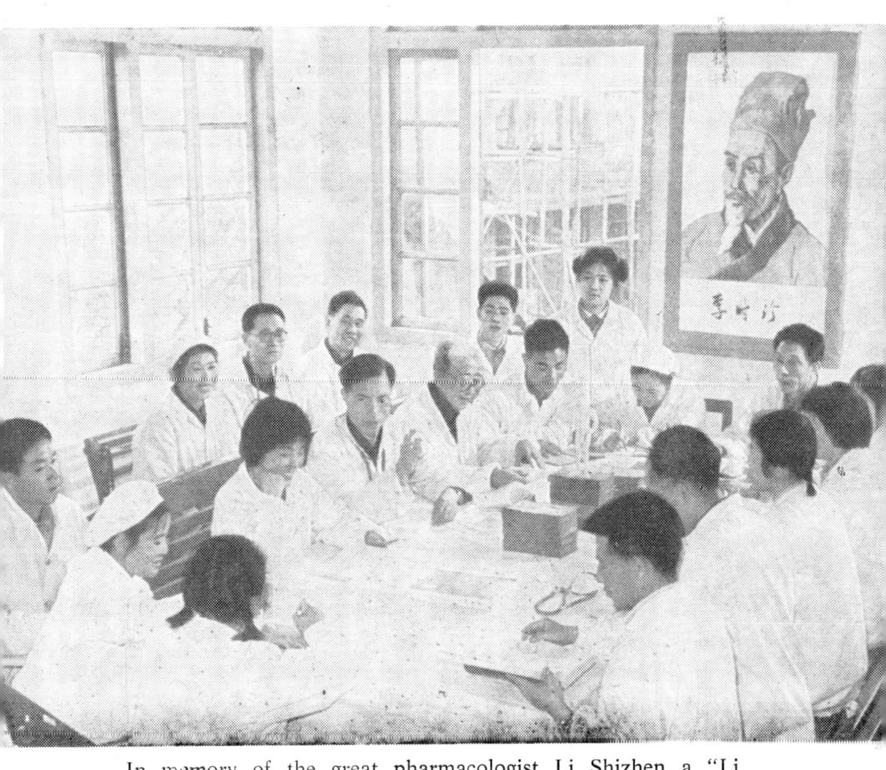

In memory of the great pharmacologist Li Shizhen, a "Li Shizhen Hospital" was built in his native place. There doctors can study traditional Chinese medicine.

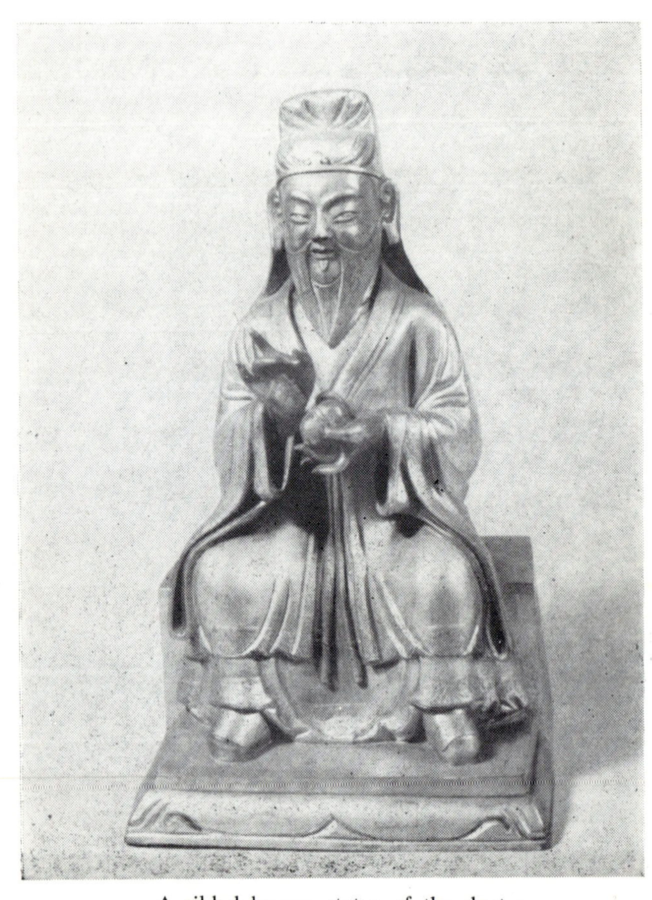

A gilded bronze statue of the doctor Sun Simiao cast in the Ming Dynasty.

PREFACE

As a cradle of one of the world's earliest civilizations, China has in the course of its historical development contributed brilliant inventions and produced many distinguished scientists, thinkers, men of letters, artists, and military strategists.

Among the remarkable cultural and scientific legacies handed down through the generations were a tremendous number of volumes on theoretical and empirical medicine and pharmacology. Traditional Chinese medicine has an important factor in improving the health of the Chinese people and bringing prosperity to the Chinese nation. It has also had a place in health care among the people of certain other countries. For several millennia Chinese medicine and pharmacology have enriched the world's knowledge in these branches of science.

The main aim of this book is to introduce the medical history of China, its achievements and evolving of an amazing system of medicine and pharmacology from ancient times. Details of clinical therapeutic methods are bypassed. The present work is written in a style of free discussion, with the desire of simply reflecting certain historical achievements in some aspects of medical science. As traditional Chinese medicine has an immense scope, the reader should understand that this volume is merely an introduction to the subject.

Here I would like to point out that owing to historical limitations and the limitations of individual medical practitioners of different eras, certain fallacies in medical theory and practice as expounded in some ancient medical works are unavoidable.

Gaps in historical data and thus in my knowledge of the subject make the work far from exhaustive, and I hope that readers will bear with this and yet find in it facts and developmental processes of interest and benefit to them.

FU WEIKANG

THE LEGENDARY SHEN NONG WHO TASTED HUNDREDS OF HERBS

A very old Chinese legend says that in the remote past there lived a certain Shen Nong, or God of Husbandry, who tasted a hundred kinds of herbs. This story was told whenever medicine and pharmacology were discussed.

According to *The Book of the Prince of Huainan*, a classic dating back 2,000 years, "Sheng Nong tasted the flavour of hundreds of herbs and drank the water from many springs and wells so that people might know which were sweet and which were bitter. On some days Shen Nong tasted as many as 70 kinds of herbs that were poisonous."

The *History of Three Emperors*, written by Sima Zhen more than 1,000 years ago, contains the passage: "Shen Nong . . . was the first man to taste hundreds of plants, bringing medicine and pharmacology into existence." So it seems that the discovery of medicinal plants came about through tasting, mainly of poisonous herbs. And it was through the tasting of herbs that people began to acquire some rudimentary medical and pharmacological knowledge.

The story about Shen Nong tasting poisonous plants is of course incredible, for no one could survive tasting seven poisonous herbs in a day, let alone 70. We may rather think then of Shen Nong as actually the embodiment of mankind's search for medicinal herbs through ages of testing, till eventually a knowledge of medicine and pharmacology evolved.

With the first herbs recognized as medicinal discovered

through the taste buds, why were the ancients motivated to "taste a hundred kinds"? An answer to this question necessitates going far back in pre-history to the life of the "Chinese ape-man".

Research done in paleontology and studies of unearthed historical relics show that as early as 1.7 million years ago the Chinese ape-man — one of the earliest human species — was alive and flourishing in the land of China.

Primitive man's productivity was extremely low and his living condition little better than that of the animals. Sheltering in caves and wearing feathers and animal skins, they had to keep constant vigil against the cruelties of nature surrounding them. They had to hide from or fight wild animals and venomous snakes. They had to search for food in the wilderness to keep themselves alive.

But what was edible and what was not? In filling their stomachs these earliest ancestors of ours were bound to try out some very disagreeable or even poisonous plants that made them itch, gave them stomach-aches and vomiting, diarrhea, or perhaps headaches. Some were certainly anesthetized or died of poisoning. Others, however, must have found relief from pain and discomfort after eating certain plants.

Through many repetitions of such experiences, pleasant or unpleasant, early man gradually learned which plants could be eaten and which caused illness, discomfort or death; also which ones relieved pain and illness. After that, people in pain sought out plants that had relieved their pain before. Such is the origin of recognizing medicinal substances, the basis of development of Chinese medicine and pharmacology.

As the natural world is most abundant in plants, it was mainly plants that primitive man sought for food, and it was therefore mainly herbs that our ancestors knew as medicinal substances.

Before the use of fire, food was eaten raw and often caused illnesses, particularly of the alimentary tract. Cooking reduced the occurrence of illness and at the same time promoted digestion and absorption of food. With the increase of food resources, the number of known edible substances grew, and drugs of animal origin were discovered. This new knowledge of medicinal substances was extended and became enriched.

In time, people learned not only to avoid poisonous substances and prevent their untoward effects. They also learned to use the poisonous substances and began to dip their arrows into them for a greater kill rate in shooting birds and beasts for food.

Primitive man inevitably suffered some injury during daily activity, and especially when hunting or during tribal infighting. They would apply such substances at hand as mud, moss or grass to their wound or bruise and dress it with leaves. Gradually they discovered that certain substances reduced swelling and relieved pain when applied externally. This primitive first-aid for traumatic injury was the origin of surgery.

The constant advance of production provided the conditions for the steady development of medicine and pharmacology. When agriculture was invented, our ancestors stopped roving and settled down to live, enabling them to observe the growth of certain plants for an extended period. This increased the range of edible plants, and with that the recognition and discovery of many more medicinal herbs.

The above shows that medicine and pharmacology developed through long-term productive labour by people in search of a richer material life. Meanwhile, medical knowledge was gaining ground through steady clinical practice.

CHINA'S EARLIEST RECORDS ON MEDICINE AND PHARMACOLOGY

Before medical and pharmacological knowledge could be preserved in written form, health hints spread from mouth to mouth and people memorized the remedies, exchanged experience, and so handed down their knowledge to later generations. With the evolution of an adequate written language, records of treatment, administraton of certain drugs and descriptions of some diseases appeared.

The earliest Chinese characters were inscriptions on ox bones and tortoise shells — actually pictographs and various signs. Since the end of the 19th century such "oracle bones" have been unearthed from the Shang Dynasty ruins in the Anyang area of Henan Province. These have been found to be 3,000 years old.

Though these bone-and-tortoise-shell inscriptions are in characters quite different from today's, having developed from primitive pictures, researchers in archaeology assure us that at that time people were already aware of disease and the importance of human hygiene. The character for "disease", for example, was symbolized by a man being shot with an arrow, looking ill and in pain. There is a picture showing a tooth with cavities and another showing intestinal parasites. Also representations of disorders of the head, ear, eye, food and so on have been found. These were the earliest characters, and also the earliest records of China's medical history.

By the Western Zhou Dynasty (c. 11th century to 771 B.C.) there was quite a collection of medical literature.

One passage in the *Rites of Zhou* (a record of the official system of the Western Zhou Dynasty court and that of various kingdoms of the Warring States Period) states that people are subject to headache in spring, scabies, boils and other skin disorders in summer, malaria in autumn and cough and asthma in winter, indicating that it was already recognized that weather is related to health and the occurrence of disease.

The *Book of Songs* compiled during the Spring and Autumn Period (770-476 B.C.), the earliest such collection in China, contains much information on gathering herbs. The medicinal herbs mentioned as being collected are plantain, fritillary, motherwort and mugwort. The therapeutic effect of these drugs is not told in the *Book of Songs*, but later medical works do discuss the action of these herbs and also other drugs of animal or herbal origin. The principal action of plantain, for instance, is described as diuretic, relieving diarrhea, clearing the eyes and dispelling sputum. The action of fritillary was to dissolve sputum and soothe cough. Motherwort was for regulating menstruation and for use as a diuretic while mugwort was the main material for moxibustion. All these herbal substances are still frequently used today.

In the ox-bone-and-tortoise-shell inscriptions appears a symbol representing the character 酒 (*jiu*, wine), indicating something very important in Chinese medicine. Very early references in Chinese literature tell of wine being used therapeutically by ancients. When tracing the source of the Chinese character 醫 (*yi*, medicine), one comes upon a fascinating story about the close relationship between medicine and wine.

According to the *Analytical Dictionary of Characters*, the earliest dictionary of the Chinese language, published in the 2nd century, the upper part of the character ("醫") is the appearance of a sick man and the lower part is the character "酒", suggesting a mode of treatment and showing the proximity of wine to medicine.

Wine has been known for a very long time; it existed in the natural environment long before it was discovered by humans. In the valleys or forests wild fruit fell to the ground when ripe, and the heat of the sun fermented it and produced fruit wine. In primitive society, when people gathered wild plants to satisfy hunger, this "fruit wine" is bound to have been ingested. Later, when people planted and also began eating cooked food, leftover cooked grain certainly fermented and became wine too. Through a long process of investigation and experimentation, people gradually learned to make wine.

The therapeutic effect of wine was in time recognized after much experimentation. Drinking a small amount of wine was found to cause excitation, while a large amount caused intoxication, with nausea and vomiting, headache, lethargy or loss of consciousness. Thus wine was said to be a drug causing excitation and anaesthesia, a rule of thumb known by people in ancient times.

When was wine first used for therapeutic purposes? Historical data at hand do not make this clear, but oracle bone inscriptions indicate that medicine was compounded with wine as early as the Shang Dynasty. Later, in the *History of the Han Dynasty*, a passage says that of all drugs, wine is the most important.

Chinese medicine claims that an appropriate amount of wine promotes blood circulation, or it may enhance the effect of drugs. In ancient times, general anaesthetic drugs were usually given by mouth and were mixed with warm wine to enhance their effect.

Since ancient days there were various kinds of famous medicated wines, such as slender acanthopanax bark wine, tiger bone wine and ginseng wine, which are still famous today.

When processing crude drugs, wine plays the important role of averting certain side effects of the substances, promoting their therapeutic effect and preserving the property of the drugs. Some drugs are first washed with wine or soaked in it; some are roasted or steamed with wine — all procedures showing the affinity of wine to medicine since ancient times.

THE FOUR DIAGNOSTIC METHODS AND EXPERIMENTAL DIAGNOSIS IN ANCIENT CHINESE MEDICINE

The four diagnostic methods in Chinese medicine are a series of basic means of recognizing disease. Gradually established since very early times through clinical practice, they are the methods of observance (observing the patient's expression, colour, appearance and tongue coating); listening and smelling (listening to the patient's voice and smelling body odour); inquiring (inquiring about the disease condition and duration, etc.); and palpation (feeling the pulse to find out its quality, power, rate, rhythm and also palpating the body for any abnormality).

The first physician to systematize and apply these four methods was Bian Que who lived around the 4th century B.C. His methods have been specially recorded by historians.

Bian Que's real name was Qin Yueren. He was born in Mozhou, Bohai Prefecture (Renqiu County in Hebei Province today). The young Bian Que worked as a steward in an inn where a famous old doctor known as Chang Sangjun lived. Bian Que was very much interested in medicine and liked to spend long hours discussing the subject with this doctor.

After a certain period of time, Chang Sangjun discovered that Bian Que was very conscientious and really wanted to learn medicine. Furthermore, he appeared to have a great sense of responsibility. Chang Sangjun therefore decided to teach him all he knew and had experienced in medicine. For 10 years Bian Que studied hard and seriously, and his medical knowledge eventually exceeded that of the elderly Chang Sang-jun, who in time died. The now prominent doctor Bian Que moreover opposed the superstition that pervaded medical practice in those days.

Although productive forces were developing and people's knowledge had broadened by the time of the Spring and Autumn Period, the superstition and preternaturalism that remained in their minds hindered the development of medical science. Bian Que was pained by this and swore to rectify all the harm done by superstition in the field of medicine. Among the six principles which Bian Que adhered to in treating his patients was discrediting all sorcery. He pointed out that patients who believed in magic power and sorcerors' supplications rather than in medicine were difficult to cure. He was not satisfied with his medical skill and was aware that what worried the doctors was their lack of methods in treating disease, while what worried the people was so much disease. To equip himself with added therapeutic techniques, he undertook the study of massage, acupuncture and moxibustion, and medicated hot compressing. To enhance the therapeutic effect, he prescribed herbal decoctions along with other kinds of treatment. He not only specialized in internal medicine but was a renowned gynaecologist and obstetrician, pediatrician and doctor of ear, nose and throat diseases.

Bian Que travelled about in his practice of medicine and treated whatever diseases afflicted the people. In Handan in present-day Hebei Province, women's diseases were prevalent, so he treated those. He treated the many ear and eye diseases he found in Luoyang, where many of the elderly were either deaf or semi-blind. He worked as a pediatrician while in Xianyang, as the children there was stricken by an endemic disease.

In diagnosis, Bian Que used the four diagnostic methods

described above, while in treatment he used multiple methods. He is said to have saved a certain Prince of Guo who had been "dead" for some time. Here is the story.

One day when Bian Que and his pupils were touring the Kingdom of Guo they heard that the prince had suddenly fallen ill and had been unconscious for half a day. People in the court thought the prince was dead and were arranging for the funeral. Bian Que doubted this and went with his pupils to investigate. Examining the prince carefully, he noted that his nostrils were moving slightly and that the skin on the inner surface of his thigh was slightly warm. He stated that the prince was not dead but in a coma. Acupuncture brought the prince around, after which herbal decoctions and hot compresses cured the prince in 20 days.

Word that Bian Que had cured the Prince of Guo so excited the people of the whole state that they said Bian Que had the power of raising the dead. Bian Que corrected this, explaining that he had not performed any such miracle, that the prince had in fact not been dead and responded to a period of treatment.

People liked Bian Que for his modesty and conscientious pursuit of knowledge. He was skilful in medicine and had the virtues of a doctor. For this, the court doctor Li Xi of the Qin Kingdom was jealous of him and had him assassinated. Yet Bian Que lived on in the hearts of the people, and the great historian Sima Qian praised him highly in his *Records of the Historian*. Even today people cherish the memory of Bian Que.

In diagnosing, modern medicine uses, in addition to the fundamental methods of inquiring, observing, palpating, percussing and auscultation, such laboratory examinations as testing the blood and urine and making bacteriological and isotomic investigations. It may be thought that such experimental procedures are of the present day only, but this is not so. As early as A.D. 752 there were methods for testing the urine of a jaundice patient, as recorded in the *Secret Prescriptions Revealed by a Provincial Governor,* published in the Tang Dynasty. The author, Wang Tao, was for a time in charge of the government Hongwen Library and so availed himself of the opportunity to read ancient Chinese literature from before the middle of the 8th century. The *Secret Prescriptions* resulted from Wang Tao's profound research into ancient Chinese medicine.

The *Secret Prescriptions* mainly discusses the symptoms and signs of various diseases and the drugs and methods to be applied in treating them. Diagnosis and moxibustion are mentioned. Mentioned twice in the book is a test of the progress of a jaundice patient. A small piece of white silk was soaked in the patient's urine every night, taken out the next day, dated and allowed to dry. The shades of colour of these pieces of silk were compared; a gradual fading of the yellow colour meant that the patient was improving, or vice versa. This is the earliest experimental clinical investigation known in the history of Chinese medicine.

Though very simple, the principle of the urine colour test still applies in some tests today — for instance, the litmus paper test. We have both quantitative and qualitative tests, and results are sometimes determined by the change in colour of a test paper. Such colour tests may aid in determining the prognosis of a disease or the therapeutic effect of treatment.

This more than 2,000-year-old method of testing the urine to determine the jaundice patient's condition, ancient and simple as it was, was innovative and a contribution to diagnosis.

THE YELLOW EMPEROR'S CANON OF MEDICINE

— First Complete Summary of Ancient Chinese Medicine

The Spring and Autumn and Warring States Period (770-221 B.C.) was a period of great social change and tremendous economic development. Iron tools came more and more into use, providing the material conditions for progress in many fields of activity. In the area of philosophy and culture, "numerous scholars came to the fore and a hundred schools of thought contended". Science, including medicine and pharmacology, flourished as never before. At that time an outstanding medical book appeared — *The Yellow Emperor's Canon of Medicine.*

Attributed to the legendary Huang Di, or Yellow Emperor, who was considered the earliest progeniter of the Chinese, the work was actually written by some unknown medical scholars of the Warring States Period. Between 221 B.C. and A.D. 220, in the dynasties of Qin and Han, other medical men made corrections and additions to the book. Thus the *Canon of Medicine* became an important classic, a complete summary of the achievements in the field of medicine before the 3rd century.

The *Canon of Medicine,* which includes the *Plain Questions* and *Vital Pivot,* expounds human anatomy, physiology, pulse, etiology, pathology, prevention of disease, diagnosis and treatment. It also discusses the relationship between man and his natural environment, and the inter-relationship of the internal organs of the human body.

Extant ancient medical books credit the *Canon of Medicine* with first using the term "anatomy". Here is one passage: "A man eight feet in height with skin and flesh can be studied externally by measuring, palpating and pressing. If he is dead, investigation can be made by anatomy of the corpse." The *Canon of Medicine* can thus be seen as fairly reliable. Moreover, much of its content is expounded in terms of such naive materialism and spontaneous dialectical concepts as the concepts that everything should be studied in relation to other things, that everything is in constant motion and change, the concept of preventive medicine and opposition to superstition. The hypotheses concerning the viscera, the channels of the body or *jing luo*,[1] the theories of *yin* and *yang*,[2] the five elements,[3] vital energy and blood, etiology, etc. discussed in the book paved the way for a theoretical system of traditional Chinese medicine.

---

1 For an explanation of *jing luo*, see pp. 87-88 below.

2 The theory of *yin* and *yang* holds that every object or phenomenon in the universe consists of two opposite aspects, namely, *yin* and *yang*, or negative and positive, which are at once in conflict and in interdependence. The theory is extensively applied in traditional Chinese medicine to explain the physiology and pathology of the human body and serve as a guide to diagnosis and treatment in clinical work.

3 The theory of the five elements holds that wood, fire, earth, metal and water are the basic materials constituting the material world. There exists among them an interdependence and inter-restraint which determines their state of constant motion and change. Its application to traditional Chinese medicine is in classifying into different categories natural phenomena plus the tissues and organs of the human body and the human emotions and interpreting the relationship between the physiology and pathology of the human body and the natural environment with the law of the inter-promoting, inter-action, over-action and counter-action of the five elements.

The *Canon of Medicine* summarizes the growth and development, maturity and the prime of life, then senility of man, giving the laws of the process. It also points out the difference in development of the male and the female.

It says that a girl starts to bloom at the age of seven, the milk teeth begin to change into permanent teeth and the hair gets thick and glossy; at the age of 14 (2×7) puberty begins and menstruation appears. When she is 21 (3×7) her growth reaches a climax, her wisdom teeth erupt. At the age of 28 (4×7) she becomes very sturdy, with strong tendons and bones. When she has passed 35 years (5×7) her bloom gradually fades and her hair starts to fall. At 42 (6×7) her face looks withered and her hair turns grey. At 49 (7×7) menopause sets in and her reproductive life is over.

As for a boy, the book says that at the age of eight he begins to grow healthy and handsome, the milk teeth change to permanent teeth and the hair becomes thick. At the age of 16 (2×8) he reaches puberty, and at 24 (3×8) his growth and development reach a climax and his wisdom teeth appear. At the age of 32 (4×8) the male becomes very sturdy, with tendons and bones tough and strong. At 40 (5 × 8) his facial glow gradually becomes dull, his hair begins to fall and his teeth lose their lustre. The age of 48 (6×8) sees his complexion withering and his hair turning grey. At 56 (7×8) the function of internal organs markedly decreases, and at 64 (8×8) as the male approaches senility, his teeth loosen and his hair thins.

Seven as the age factor for the female and eight for the male in the process of human growth was an ancient Chinese deduction after numerous observations. Obviously, the life span was much shorter and senility set in earlier then than now, due to the poor living conditions at that time. The saying, "For a man to reach 70 years of age has been rare since ancient times," reflects this. Still the *Canon of Medicine* expounds the developmental process of men and women, and their senility, basically outlining the contemporary picture.

As for human physiological organic function, descriptions in the *Canon* are not far off. "The head is the domicile of wisdom and thought," e.g., refers to the brain. That the brain and spinal cord are vital organs not to be acupunctured is stressed, recognizing the vulnerability of these organs. The book points out that any accidental needling in that area could cause death or serious damage to the spinal cord.

Numerous descriptions involving human blood circulation, the heart and vascular system in the *Canon of Medicine* are surprisingly accurate. It says: "The heart is the foundation of life"; "The heart dominates the body's blood vessels"; "The blood in all vessels flows to the heart," showing early recognition of the importance of the heart, in close contact with the blood vessels.

Its views on vascular function and the blood are also correct in considering the blood vessels on the one hand as being the passageways for blood circulation, and on the other as transport lines for nutrition to the nerves, bones, muscles and viscera of the whole body. Blood contains the various nutritional substances which it carries to supply the entire body for promoting the normal activity of its various parts. The *Canon* says, for instance, "When the liver is filled with blood, then the person can see; if the feet flow with blood, then he can walk. If the palm and fingers are nourished with blood, the hand can hold things and the fingers can flex." These observations reflect scientific facts.

Modern science makes a clear distinction between the components of the blood in the arteries and in the veins. The *Canon of Medicine* points out as early as 2,000 years ago that when one kind of vessel is punctured, blood spurts out and its colour is bright red. From another kind of vessel the blood does not spurt, and its colour is dull and turbid. However, this could not be well explained at that time.

Change in pulse rate is also observed then as reflecting a person's emotions, physiology and pathology. Quoting again from the *Canon*, "When a person is frightened, fatigued, under stress or at rest, the pulse is different." From there, based on prolonged clinical practice, Chinese medical practitioners gradually formulated the theory of diagnosis by pulse-taking.

The blood in the human body, which contains a certain kind of gaseous and nutritional substance, flows to and converges in various parts of the body through the heart and the vascular system, with the heart as centre. Blood forms a circulatory system which flows endlessly. A passage in the *Canon* says, "The blood flows in the vessels unceasingly and it circulates in the body endlessly" — an obviously correct understanding.

The *Canon* also makes a number of correct remarks on respiration, digestion, excretion and motion. For example, it mentions specifically the relationship among perspiration, body temperature and urination. It comments that profuse perspiration may lower temperature in hot weather; in cold weather there is less perspiration and so urination is more frequent.

Although there are various internal organs with different structures and functions in the human body, these organs are not independent of each other, says the *Canon*. On the contrary they control and influence each other and are in organic co-operation, carrying out the biological activities of the human body. This view in the *Canon* is based on the concept of viewing things as mutually related, that is to say, viewing the human body in relation to the natural environment, each organ in relation to the other organs and each part of the body in relation to the whole body.

The *Canon of Medicine* holds that normal physiological activity can only be maintained when a relative balance is kept among various internal organs, and between these organs and the external environment. Once this balance and co-ordination is lost, disease sets in.

The *Canon* also attaches great importance to the normal and healthy functioning of the internal organs of the body, considering this an essential factor. It says that if the vital functions and resistance of the human body are normal and full, then exopathogenic factors (harmful agents) have no avenue to invade, or will not necessarily cause illness. Conversely, invasion by exopathogenic factors is possible when internal function becomes abnormal and body resistance is low.

The *Canon* thus says: "All types of disease may occur when one is over-exposed to wind, rain, cold or heat; also when there is imbalance of *yin* and *yang*; or in extreme joy or anger, with irregular eating, undesirable living conditions, or in a state of fright or dread." Though bacteria were not recognized as disease factors, nervous tension, anxiety, sudden violent change of emotion, improper food and abnormal change of environmental conditions were recognized as factors leading to disease. This understanding countered the view at that time that diseases were due to devils or punishment by gods.

The naive materialist views of the Warring States Period were applied in the *Canon* to its refutation of mysticism and superstition. One chapter comments: "It is no use to talk about medical principles with persons who believe in ghosts and spirits; neither is there any way to discuss medical techniques with persons who oppose acupuncture, surgery and medicinal substances."

The *Canon* goes deeply into many diseases. It first describes briefly infectious diseases which are very harmful to human beings, saying: "When infectious diseases prevail, they may pass from one person to another, whether adults or children, the symptoms and signs being the same."

A special chapter on malaria mentions the tertian, quartan, and the malignant quotidian types of malaria.

As to jaundice, edema due to nephritis, malnutrition, anaemia and other diseases, the book is quite accurate too. It observes that in nephritis edema usually appears in the eyelids. It records that whenever a hailstorm occurred the crops were badly affected and most of the people suffered from perleche. Perhaps in modern medical terms this would be a lack of riboflavin. As to symptoms of anaemia and loss of blood, the *Canon* stresses facial pallor and lack of lustre.

The *Canon of Medicine* also discusses cough, diarrhea, bloody stool, abscess, swollen throat, swelling of the lymph nodes of the neck, cholera, hemorrhoids, arthritis, epilepsy, etc., about 300 diseases and symptoms in all. These were diagnosed through the methods of observation, listening and smelling, inquiring and feeling the pulse.

In curing disease, the *Canon* emphasizes prevention and early treatment, claiming that only those doctors who practise in this way are good doctors.

This book claims that the state of health and occurrence of disease in each individual are different due to differences in environmental climate and customs, and that methods of treatment should therefore be different. Therapeutic measures include acupuncture, massage, hot compresses, physical exercise and drugs.

The *Canon* is an optimistic book. It says that all kinds of disease are curable. One chapter is devoted to four parables to put the idea across. It says disease can be compared to being pricked with a thorn, or the skin being soiled, a string knotted or a river obstructed. But the thorn can be removed, the dirt can be washed away, the knot can be untied, the obstruction cleared. That man can "conquer nature" and cure every disease is a prospect for the future, when doctors have grasped the methods, techniques and measures to take. Much is still unknown in curing disease, but the idea that every disease has its cure is a strong refutation of any such concept as fate governing our lives and health.

In short, the *Canon of Medicine* is a Chinese medical classic rich in content. It is the most outstanding of the four famous Chinese medical classics. It not only laid the foundation for formulating the distinctive system of ancient Chinese medical theory but also contributed greatly towards the development of Chinese medicine. Moreover, the book was known abroad as early as 1,400 years ago. A medical history of Japan says, for example, that a medical college of Japan was using the *Canon of Medicine* as one of its main textbooks in A.D. 701.[1]

---

[1] Fujikawa Yu, *The Medical History of Japan,* Tokyo, 1941.

SHEN NONG'S CANON OF HERBS

— Earliest Extant Book on Chinese Pharmacology

The earliest extant Chinese book specializing in pharmacology is the *Shen Nong's Canon of Herbs*, known also as the *Canon of Herbs*, written in the 1st and 2nd centuries.

In traditional Chinese medicine the term "herbs" means Chinese drugs, because herbs are the basic material used in treating disease, although medicines of animal or mineral origin are also used.

The term "herb" first appeared around the 1st century or a little earlier in the "Record of Sacrifice" of the *History of the Han Dynasty* which points out: "In the second year of the Emperor Cheng Di of the Han Dynasty [31 B.C.], 70 officials were dismissed and sent back to their hometowns, including those in charge of medicine and herbs."

The writer of the *Canon of Herbs* is unknown, but as the ancient people were greatly influenced by the legend of Shen Nong who tasted hundreds of herbs, they ascribed the book to him. Actually the book summarizes experience in using the drugs of our forefathers before the Han Dynasty.

The *Canon of Herbs* lists 365 medicinal substances, 252 of which are of plant origin, while 67 kinds are of animal origin and 46 of mineral.

The *Canon of Herbs* briefly describes the places where drugs are produced, their synonyms, properties and indications.

The preface of the book gives a preliminary summary of the basic theory of some of the drugs' uses, detailing the administration of a single drug, and in a compound prescription how to co-ordinate the main and the adjuvant drugs, and the combined prescriptions. Contraindications are also mentioned.

The effects of the herbs depend on the region of production, season of collection and method of preparation. Some herbs require drying in the sun, some should be dried slowly in a shady place; some are suitable to make into pills, others are suitable for powder. Some should be boiled in water, while others should be soaked or roasted in wine. Certain herbs must not be prepared with wine. The *Canon of Herbs* explains these methods in detail and also explains how to identify the herbal substances morphologically.

The *Canon of Herbs* also advises on dosage, especially of toxic drugs. Small doses are suggested to begin with, then increased gradually if the reaction is good.

Most medicinal substances recorded in the *Canon of Herbs* have genuine therapeutic effect, and many are still used today. Chinese jujube and angelica are still taken as tonics; the tuber of pinellia and polygala root resolve sputum; the root of balloonflower and almond suppress cough and pacify asthma; peppermint clears the mind; salvia root relieves pain; honey is laxative; rhubarb is purgative; plantain produces diuresis; ephedra soothes asthma; coptis checks bacterial dysentery, the root of antipyretic lichroa is used in treating malaria; seaweed is used for goiter, realgar as insecticide. Modern science confirms the above-mentioned drugs as appropriate remedies for the specified diseases. The names and symptoms of diseases as recorded in the *Canon of Herbs* give a partial understanding of pathology in older times.

It is little wonder that the *Canon of Herbs* is listed by succeeding generations as one of the four famous Chinese medical classics, and is highly significant in medical history, as it was the first work to summarize Chinese medicinal herbs and so laid the foundation for developing Chinese pharmacology.

TREATISE ON FEBRILE AND OTHER DISEASES
— the First Chinese Medical Book on Clinical Therapy and Diagnosis

The *Treatise on Febrile and Other Diseases* was written by the outstanding physician Zhang Zhongjing in about A.D. 210. It is the first important work on clinical therapy and diagnosis that has come down to us.

Zhang Zhongjing lived around the middle of the 2nd century to the second decade of the 3rd century, at the end of the Eastern Han Dynasty.

Epidemics plagued the people and claimed many lives in various places in China in the Han Dynasty. Before the first year of the Jianan reign (A.D. 196), Zhang Zhongjing's clan numbered more than 200 people, of whom two-thirds died within 10 years, 70 per cent of infectious diseases. Zhang Zhongjing thus commented on seeing his clan members perish one after another: "To think of the death in the present and past! How can one let such disaster continue? A way must be found to save the people, and the way is to look into ancient teachings and gather together all available prescriptions."

After unremitting efforts he drew on and summarized the medical achievements of his forerunners, and combining these with his own clinical practice he wrote the *Treatise on Febrile and Other Diseases* which includes Chinese medical theory. His work was a noteworthy contribution to clinical diagnosis and treatment.

As printing had not yet been invented, the *Treatise on Febrile and Other Diseases* was copied by hand and the copies were circulated. These were mostly lost in subsequent wars, but the work was afterwards retrieved, and at the end of the 3rd century the physician Wang Shuhe organized and edited the book, bits of which he had arduously collected. In the 11th century, Lin Yi recompiled the book, dividing it into the *Treatise on Febrile Diseases* and *Jingui Collection of Prescriptions* and had it published. It is in this 11th-century form that we are still using it today.

The *Treatise on Febrile Diseases* describes the symptoms and signs of various acute febrile diseases, including typhoid, typhus, cholera and dysentery, and their diagnoses and therapeutic methods. It also mentions the common cold, influenza, pneumonia, purulent pneumonia, tetanus, enteritis and what we know today as encephalitis and appendicitis. Based on the channel theory of Chinese medicine, Zhang Zhongjing deducted six syndromes from the viewpoint of six pairs of channels in the human body to explain the rules of exopathological factor invasion when changes occur in the natural environment such as a change in weather bringing on epidemic disease. He listed the main and secondary symptoms and signs, and then proposed corresponding general and specific treatment according to the patient's state of health and the symptoms and signs, reflecting the principle of flexibility in treatment.

The *Jingui Collection of Prescriptions* mainly describes "miscellaneous diseases" according to the traditional Chinese medical theory of the viscera. It differentiates and classifies diseases and gives their causes, including internal functional changes, invasion of the body by exopathological factors, or injury by an outside force. It describes diabetes as a disease of "three excessives" — excessive eating, excessive drinking and excessive urination — a picture in conformity with today's knowledge of diabetes.

Artificial respiration is prescribed as an emergency measure for patients who have stopped breathing. The *Jingui Collection* comments on the procedure: " . . . One should press with the hands on the patient's chest with rapid movements." This technique is roughly what is used today. It is also a method of cardiac massage.

Another important contribution of Zhang Zhongjing was introducing the science of combining drugs. While the *Canon of Medicine* lists only 12 prescriptions and 5 forms of drugs — decoction, tincture, pills, powder and pellet, the *Treatise on Febrile Diseases* and *Jingui Collection* give 370 prescriptions and a greater variety of forms including emulsion. There are also directions for washing, soaking, fumigating, using ear and nose drops, nasal and anal drug administration and applying ointments and suppositories. The *Jingui Colection* prescribes alum pills (mixture of alum and almond) to treat leukorrhia, the earliest reference to a gynecological suppository still adapted for use today. For his contribution to traditional Chinese pharmacology, Zhang Zhongjing became known as "Father of Prescriptions" from the Han Dynasty, when he lived.

Prescriptions mentioned in the *Treatise on Febrile and Other Diseases* for treating dysentery, B-type encephalitis, pneumonia, hepatitis and appendicitis are still applicable today, having been studied and improved to obtain good clinical results. The book also introduces "smoked plum pills" for treating the vomiting of worms. These pills are still useful in treating ascariasis of the bile duct.

Zhang Zhongjing in his *Treatise* refuted superstition and quackery, sharply criticizing advocates of mysticism in the face of disease who did not pay attention to medical treatment. What such quacks pursue is wealth and fame, he said, and once disease threatens they panic and resort to sorcery. When death occurred, they would say it was "fate", that the mortality was foreordained.

Zhang Zhongjing believed that when death set in, the person's spirit and mental activity stopped and the body became another substance.

Zhang also focused attention on learning from other doctors and opposed one-sided views and such conservative ideas as "family secret skill" and "clinging to the old". He berated being guided by the appearance of things and neglecting their essence, saying: "Things that look magnificent may be rotten inside." Attaching importance to early treatment, he said that disease could become stubborn and difficult to handle if not treated in time, especially diseases of women and children.

As to hygiene and food, the *Jingui Collection* advises against eating anything that is stale or spoiled, fruit that has been contaminated by flies and insects, and the meat of dead animals, whether ox, sheep or pig.

The *Treatise on Febrile Diseases* and *Jingui Collection of Prescriptions* are the two most influential books in the field in China after the *Canon of Medicine.* They summarized medical theory, treatment methods, and combining and prescribing drugs. The works further established the principle of differentiating disease according to individual symptoms and signs. They are two of the four best-known ancient texts which are required reading for students of traditional Chinese medicine. Taken as guides in clinical treatment, they have found use also in Korea and Japan.

HANDBOOK FOR EMERGENCIES

— Ancient Manual on Treatment in Emergencies

Ge Hong (c. A.D. 284-364) wrote the *Handbook for Emergencies* and had it published 1,600 years ago.

The medicaments prescribed in this book were substances either at hand or easily available and relatively inexpensive. In his preface, Ge Hong criticizes writers of books for emergencies who were themselves unable even briefly to describe the nature of the attack, and who prescribed drugs beyond the reach of peasants' purses. Ge Hong kept three things in mind: therapeutic effect, availability, and cost.

Diseases mentioned in the *Handbook for Emergencies* include such infectious and parasitic diseases as tuberculosis, cholera, typhoid, malaria and intestinal parasitosis; malnutrition; gastrointestinal diseases, such as choking and food poisoning; such neurological symptoms as epilepsy and mania; and surgical and dermatological conditions involving abscesses, ulcers, animal bites, boils and skin diseases. Intoxication by medicine or alcohol, swallowing foreign bodies, drowning, baldness; ear, nose, throat diseases; cough, apoplexy, coma, edema, jaundice and backache are all dealt with.

The *Handbook for Emergencies* describes in detail the complex nature, symptoms and signs of tuberculosis: The patient is usually afraid of cold, and has fever, poor appetite, restlessness, depression and general malaise, but no specific pain. The illness is lingering and wasting; and the patient becomes dull and exhausted, and dies. The *Handbook* says that tuberculosis is an infectious disease which may spread to the patients' whole family, and that a man is liable to contract the disease after a long period of overwork or when he has not recovered from prolonged illness. The *Handbook* points out that people living in south China are susceptible to beriberi. The patient is described as feeling slight pain and numbness in the lower extremities at onset, after which they become swollen and weak, and standing and walking become difficult. In the more serious form of the disease, the patient has distention of the lower abdomen and becomes dull. If this is not treated in time, there may be palpitation and shortness of breath, and death may ensue. It warns of cardiac involvement. Soyabeans, peas and milk are recommended for treatment, foods recognized today as containing readily absorbable vitamin B. This is the earliest detailed record in China of beriberi.

The *Handbook* also says of leprosy that at first the patient feels numbness of the skin, or an itchy feeling like insects creeping. It points out that the disease is serious and that the patient should be isolated.

The *Handbook* describes jaundice thus: the patient's cornea is at first yellow, then the colouring is generalized. The urine should be examined as well, to aid in diagnosis. This was done by asking the patient to urinate on a piece of white paper and noting the colour.

First mentioned in this book is dealing with such emergencies as stroke, coma and sudden abdominal attacks. For resuscitation, it prescribes pressing the philtrum (Point Renzhong) with the nail, or applying moxibustion at Point Chengjiang on the lower lip; for coma, pinellia is ground into powder and blown into the patient's nose, or dry calamus is ground and made into pills half the size of a date stone to place under the patient's tongue. These methods are still found to be effective.

That patients with edema or ascites should be wary of salt is common knowledge today. Yet the *Handbook* already cited this caution, and advised the intake of rice with red beans, bean milk and mussels. Mutton, poultry and egg yolks are mentioned as being rich in nourishment.

Preventive medicine is also reflected in the *Hanbdook* in reference to treating epidemic and febrile diseases. It says that during an epidemic, every member of the family should take preventive medicine regularly to help ward off the disease.

Besides medication, acupuncture and massage, the *Handbook for Emergencies* talks about cold and hot compresses. Its pages introduce and quote medical literature written before the 4th century, some of which was subsequently lost, and so this book has preserved certain valuable records from ancient times.

The *Handbook for Emergencies* stresses successful practical experience, and its title reflects this attitude, eschewing such highflown names as "Yellow Emperor" and "God of Husbandry". Ge Hong says in his preface: "Nowadays people generally revere the past to the neglect of the present, worship the old and despise the new. If my book is not acceptable to them because I have not attributed the prescriptions to ancient sages, well, I cannot force it on them." Such was Ge Hong's popular view of the medical profession.

"DRAGON GATE PRESCRIPTIONS"

— Ancient Recipes Engraved on Stone

Ancient Chinese prescriptions were hand-copied for circulation and reference by later generations before the invention of block printing, after which they were handed down in print. There were also more permanent prescriptions engraved on stone for what the ancients considered would be eternal preservation. The sites chosen were places frequented by many people, such as scenic spots.

Engraving in stone, however, involving much labour, necessarily limited the number of prescriptions so preserved, not to mention their destruction by weathering and other factors, so that few remain today.

The earliest extant stone-engraving recipes are the anonymous Dragon Gate Prescriptions executed 1,400 years ago. Their title derives from their being carved in a cave at Dragon Gate, 12 kilometres south of Luoyang in Henan Province. The cave was called Dragon Gate Prescriptions Cave from the time of the carving at the end of the 5th century after the Northern Wei Dynasty established its capital there. Carving at Luoyang continued over a period of some 400 years. Extant are 1,300 stone caves containing some 100,000 Buddha images.

Dragon Gate Prescriptions Cave had carved in it about 100 prescriptions from the sixth year of the Wuping period of the Northern Qi (A.D. 575) to the Tang Dynasty (A.D. 618-907). Though weather-worn over the centuries, some of the characters are still legible, and these are records of three types of therapeutic methods: prescriptions, acupuncture and moxibustion, and combining drugs with acupuncture. Among the prescriptions are herbal remedies for malaria, indigestion, vomiting, angina pectoris, allergy, fishbone in the throat and laryngitis.

Most of the prescriptions are a single drug, perhaps two, but seldom more. For malaria, for example, the single drug *Dichroa febifuga* is prescribed, and it is specified that the drug should be taken with wine before an attack.

For allergy it says that the affected area should be bathed in water boiled with willow branches; for dysentery, the juice of *Annabis savitiva* boiled with mung beans should be drunk on an empty stomach; moxibustion is recommended for fistula, the fuming material being croton and moxa, or sulphur and moxa.

It can be seen from the above that though the prescriptions were few and simple, most were effective and became popular remedies. Dragon Gate Prescriptions are valuable today for research into pharmaceuticals before the 7th century.

EARLIEST GOVERNMENT-SPONSORED MEDICAL SCHOOL AND PHARMACOPOEIA

This first government medical academy is significant because in ancient China, before the Han Dynasty, physicians and pharmacologists obtained their knowledge mainly from their forebears or as apprentices of experienced persons in the field. It was during the Southern and Northern Dynasties era, in A.D. 443, that the emperor's physician, Qin Chengzu, proposed the setting up of a medical school to be run by the state. This was done, but in A.D. 453, less than a decade later, the project ended.

In A.D. 581, in the Sui Dynasty, an Imperial Medical Academy was established. This high-level medical institution, also organized by the state, undertook certain clinical functions and had on its staff instructors in medicine and pharmacology, physicians and administrators.

In the year 624, six years after the Tang Dynasty succeeded the Sui, the Tang court established its Imperial Medical Academy on a still larger scale, with departments and faculties and a clearly defined curriculum. The departments of medicine and pharmacology were further divided into sections. Medicine included internal medicine, acupuncture, massage and incantation (the last was due to the fact that Buddhism and Taoism were prevalent at the time). Each of these specialities was headed by a person with recognized qualifications who was charged with the instruction.

Headed by these medical specialists, the staff of each section varied; e.g., internal medicine had assistants, clinical physicians and helpers. Acupuncture had assistants, acupuncturists and helpers. Masseurs and helpers staffed the massage section. Staff size varied as well, but all sections did both academic and clinical work.

Terms of training varied also. Internal medicine took seven years, surgery and pediatrics both five, ear, nose, throat and stomatology four years, cupping etc. three years. Required reading and courses included *The Yellow Emperor's Canon of Medicine,* pharmacology, the *Canon of Acupuncture and Moxibustion* and the *Classic on Pulse.* Specialities were taken up after these basic courses were completed.

Students were given regular examinations each month, term and end of year. The monthly exams were presided over by professors, term exams by imperial doctors, and annual exams by the highest imperial consultant. Students were appraised on the basis of these written examinations plus the results of their clinical practice. Those graduating with distinction were selected for responsible posts.

The Tang Dynasty department of pharmacology had a herb garden covering 18 hectares, and students known as "herb gardeners" were commoners enrolled between the ages of 16 and 20. Their main courses were identification of herb species, their cultivation, collection, storage, and points for attention in combining herbs and contraindications in prescribing drugs. Upon graduation these herb gardeners were responsible for cultivating fresh herbs for timely treatment when necessary. They also collected special herbs from various regions — the so-called natural drugs.

True, the Imperial Medical Academy was established to serve only the ruling class, yet its specialized departments and sections, assignment of instructors and staff, curricula, years of training and examination system were unprecedented.

* * *

During the early part of the 7th century after the beginning of the Tang Dynasty, the pharmaceutical book that circulated among the people was the *Canon of Herbs with Annotations,* which was compiled by Tao Hongjing from the end of the 5th century to the beginning of the 6th.

Tao Hongjing was a native of south China and his medical knowledge and use of medicinal herbs were necessarily limited to that area. Though the *Canon of Herbs with Annotations* discusses 730 kinds of herbs, very few were from the north. There were also errors in the book. But herbal medicine developed nonetheless, new drugs were discovered. China, which had further been united by the Tang Dynasty, developed communication within the country and abroad, and this promoted the interchange of pharmaceutical knowledge.

In A.D. 657 the pharmacologist Su Jing felt the necessity of compiling a new book on herbs and proposed this to the Tang court which at that time focused great attention on culture and science and so accepted the proposal without delay.

The Tang government appointed Su Jing, Xu Jingzong, Lü Cai and others, altogether 20-some-odd people, to make the compilation. Most were herbal experts, some meteorologists, while others were librarians with a knowledge of literature. With such a team the editing work would be smooth.

So that the book should include all medicinal substances of the entire country the Tang government ordered every prefecture and district to report the herbs of their area with illustrations and submit these to the capital, at that time Chang'an (present-day Xi'an). Taking the *Canon of Herbs with Annotations* as a basis, the compilers would complete the book with local material. After two years of work, in the year 659, the *Revised Canon of Herbs* was finally published and distributed throughout the whole country. This revised pharmacopoeia was the first in the history of Chinese medicine to be published by the government.

As Su Jing, Lü Cai and the others had a great rejuvenating spirit, they put great effort into collecting and sorting material for the *Revised Canon of Herbs.* Useful herbs not listed in the *Shen Nong's Canon of Herbs* were added; on the contrary, some herbs listed in certain books by popular doctors but of uncertain therapeutic value were omitted. Su Jing and his team therefore enquired extensively concerning herbs and carefully observed experience in their use among the people. The *Revised Canon of Herbs* points out the importance of regional source and season of collection to their therapeutic effect. It says that change of weather affected the nature of the herbs. This 7th-century pharmacopoeia, summing up Chinese pharmaceuticals at the time, has high scientific value.

The 54 volumes of the *Revised Canon of Herbs* appeared in three parts: Botany, Illustrations, and Captions. Botany includes descriptions of the properties, flavour and characteristics of the herbs, their source, method of collection, important points for attention, and therapeutic effect. A total of 844 herbs are included in the book, over 100 more than that in the *Canon of Herbs with Annotations.* Among the newly added species are such highly effective drugs as castor bean, dandelion and also some drugs introduced from foreign lands.

Moreover, tin, silver and mercury are mentioned in the book in connection with dentistry and the filling of teeth — the earliest record in this branch of medicine.

The *Revised Canon of Herbs* influenced the study and practice of pharmacology for 300 years, and was circulated abroad. In the year 731 a hand-copied edition of the work appeared in Japan. It had been copied by Tanabe Fubito, who had studied in China. At the beginning of the 10th century the Japanese work *Engishiki* points out that "every doctor reads the *Revised Canon of Herbs* edited by Su Jing".

It is regrettable that the illustrations and captions of this book were lost during the Song Dynasty. A hand-copied edition of the Botany part was later found in the Dunhuang Caves in Gansu. But in the early part of the 20th century, it was stolen by foreign adventurers along with numerous other treasures stored in these caves. Fragments of this book are now stored in the British Museum and the Bibliothèque Nationale in Paris. The incomplete copy in China today was photogravured from the one hand-copied by Tanabe Fubito and preserved in Japan.

GOLDEN PRESCRIPTIONS FOR EMERGENCIES AND *SUPPLEMENTARY GOLDEN PRESCRIPTIONS*

During the 7th century medical books appeared in China with titles embellished with "golden". Two of these were the *Golden Prescriptions for Emergencies* and *Supplementary Golden Prescriptions* written by the famous doctor Sun Simiao. Why "golden"? Sun Simiao said: "A human life is the most precious thing. A physician's duty is to give his patients the best possible care." Later generations referred to these two works as the *Golden Prescriptions.*

Sun Simiao (581-682), a native of Huayuan in what is today's Yaoxian County, Shaanxi Province, made a great contribution to medicine through summarizing past medical achievements and developing his own creative ability. Besides practising medicine, Sun Simiao engaged in research and compiled pre-7th century medical literature. Among his original works were the *Golden Prescriptions for Emergencies* and *Supplementary Golden Prescriptions,* each of which consists of 30 volumes.

Sun Simiao maintained that since a physician's work directly affects his patients' health and lives, he should be of noble character and proficient in his work. He should read broadly to gain comprehensive knowledge for a firm foundation in treating disease. He observed that diseases were very complicated, and that certain diseases have similar internal symptoms but different external ones and vice versa.

Sun Simiao urged that a doctor should be vigorous and attentive, should treat patients with discretion and calm, examining them carefully, and contemplating each case deeply; he should not talk unnecessarily, make critical remarks about other doctors or over-estimate his own capabilities. He emphasized that a doctor should be sympathetic with the patient and care for him with great responsibility and that in front of the patient, one should not balk at filthiness or fetid smells. If there are difficult or emergency cases, one should never discriminate rich from poor, old from young, attractive from unappealing, but treat every patient with equality. One should not fear hardship, take cases both in daytime and at night, in severe cold and extremely hot weather, disregard hunger, thirst and fatigue, and always think out a way to rescue the patient whole-heartedly.

Besides attaching great importance to the character of a doctor, Sun Simiao contributed greatly to various aspects of medicine. In his books he gave detailed descriptions concerning prevention of diseases, diagnosis, medicinal substances, planning prescriptions, acupuncture and dietetic treatment. He paid special attention to the peculiarities of women and children, even arranging gynecology and pediatrics in front of other specialities in his book.

Sun Simiao provided valuable views and experience on the etiology and treatment of some diseases. He said that "the disease factor in cholera is due to improper food and not to the devil or any god". He introduced the experience of treating night blindness with goat or ox liver. Modern science proves that livers of animals are rich in vitamin A and can alleviate night blindness, which is mostly due to a deficiency in vitamin A. He also mentioned that swelling of the thyroid glands could be treated by ingesting the thyroid of the sheep or deer. It is now known that the thyroid glands of animals are rich in iodine, which is a genuinely effective treatment for patients deficient in iodine. As to the diet of patients with edema, Sun Simiao advised that they should beware of eating much salt.

In pharmacology Sun Simiao also made an outstanding contribution. He stressed that herbs should be collected at the proper time, and methods of processing should be correct. So in his book he mentioned the proper gathering time for 230 kinds of herbs, and advised people to gather them during the right season and preserve them for emergency use. Sun was called the "King of Herbs" by later generations because of his extraordinary contributions to pharmacology. In his native place, a hill was call the "Hill of the King of Herbs".

It was no accident that Sun Simiao made such important achievements. He studied and worked very hard since childhood, reading extensively and intensively. At the age of seven he could recite 1,000 words a day. On the other hand he was not healthy and often fell ill when young, so that his parents had to call for a doctor and buy drugs. Because of this, their resources became strained. At the same time he became aware of the pain of his relatives and neighbours when they were sick, so he began to study medicine and pharmacology from his youth. Based on his studies, he treated himself and eventually recovered his health. Sometimes he treated his relatives and neighbours when they were ill, with good results.

Sun Simiao became much renowned for his knowledge and profound medical erudition. Emperors Wendi of the Sui Dynasty and Emperors Taizong and Gaozong of the Tang Dynasty successively invited him to their courts. He refused, as he was not seeking money or fame and preferred to serve his own patients. In the old society, such noble gestures of refusing personal glory and wealth were rare and admirable.

After the publication of the *Golden Prescriptions for Emergencies* and *Supplementary Golden Prescriptions,* these two books profoundly influenced the medicine of later generations. Many Chinese medical books after the 8th century quoted from them. In the year 1124, Guo Si, based on the contents of the two books, wrote the *Important Golden Prescriptions* which was engraved on stone at Huazhou. Sun Simiao's books also greatly influenced medical science abroad, as we know from the 10th-century *Prescriptions for Treating the Heart* written by the Japanese Nima Yasunori, which cited Sun Simiao's works as references. In the 15th century, the Koreans Jin Li-Mong and others compiled the *Categories of Prescriptions*, a series of medical books which had also absorbed some of the contents of Sun Simiao's great works.

In 1961, the 1380th anniversary of the birth of Sun Simiao, the Ministry of Posts and Telecommunications of China issued commemorative stamps for the occasion showing China's continued esteem for him.

COMPENDIUM OF MATERIA MEDICA

— A Major Pharmacopoeia of the 16th Century

The *Compendium of Materia Medica* is a great work written by Li Shizhen, the world famous pharmacologist and physician. The book consists of about 1,900,000 characters, lists 1,800 kinds of drugs, and includes 1,100 illustrations and 11,000 recipes. It was the result of 27 years of hard work.

Li Shizhen (1518-93) was born into a poor family, his father a highly experienced folk doctor. Because in the feudal society, a folk doctor held a low social status, his father did not want Li to follow in his footsteps. Instead of experiencing the insolence of society, he wanted his son to take the imperial examinations. Li Shizhen, however, failed in the examinations. Since as a child he had always followed his father in collecting herbs, accompanied him to treat the ill, copied prescriptions and developed a profound sympathy for the patients, he became determined to practise medicine among the people too.

Through clinical practice, Li found that existing pharmaceutical books were full of errors, with some species incorrectly identified and confusion in the names. He resolved to go over the books thoroughly, revise them and compile a new pharmaceutical book which would be more practical.

To achieve a deeper understanding of the different kinds of herbs, their cultivation, morphology, properties, proper collection times, methods of processing and their therapeutic results, Li went into the wilderness and mountains. He meekly sought wisdom from the farmers, herb collectors, medicinal workers, wood cutters, hunters and fishermen. He planted some of the herbs himself, tasted them and made experiments. For instance, in order to verify the assertion made by previous generations that pangolins opened their scales to tempt the ants to come, and afterwards ate them, he observed the pangolins himself, discovering that they threw out their tongues to tempt the ants and then ate them. He dissected the pangolins and found that their stomachs were full of ants. To find out whether datura had the anesthetic effect which ancient books mentioned, Li took the herb himself and proved that it was true.

Li Shizhen's continuous contact with the working people and his attention to practical work resulted in the optimistic philosophy: "Man is able to overcome nature." He was convinced that man is able to learn nature's laws and use these laws for his own end. He also believed: "People are able to develop the achievements of their predecessors and discover what they had not."

Thus Li Shizhen was able to make the *Compendium of Materia Medica* practical, valuable and scientific. Nowadays we use distilled essence of honeysuckle for an antipyretic in the summer with an anti-bacterial effect. Li Shizhen made minute observations of the flower and discovered that when budding the flowers are white, though when they open after two or three days they turn yellow. He said that the new blossoms together with the old blossoms formed the colour of white and gold, and so honeysuckle was also called the gold and silver flower.

For those herbs similar in shapes and hence likely to be confused, Li stressed that "they should be collected one by one and studied minutely so as to find out their real nature". The leaves of the "Chicken Intestine Grass" and that of the "Goose Intestine Grass" looked very much the same, for instance. But when he experimented on them, Li discovered that when chewing the former plant raw the mouth would salivate smoothly, while when chewing the latter, no saliva would flow at all. This proved that Li had chewed these two kinds of herbs and identified them by noting the saliva produced in the mouth.

Li knew how to plan a prescription according to symptoms and signs and always built his recommendations on the experience of his forerunners. Once the imperial concubine of Prince Jingmu was suffering from severe gastralgia. Many doctors had been consulted but in vain. They gave her an emetic, carminatives and digestives, but she would vomit as soon as each drug was put into her mouth. There was no way to make her swallow, and the patients had not moved her bowels for three days. Li remembered that in one of the classics it said that *Corydalis yanhusuo* was able to give immediate relief of severe gastric pain. So he prescribed 0.3 ounces of the drug and made her take it with warm wine. The pain soon vanished and the constipation was relieved, exactly the desired effect. Pharmaceutical analysis tells us that it was the alkaloid *yanhusuo* in the drug which produced the analgesic effect; that substance also promotes blood circulation and removes blood stasis.

In the *Materia Medica,* Li Shizhen had written much that revealed how he and the masses together discovered new herbs and new views. Li was the first to make a detailed record and work out the exact properties of *Gynura segetum,* the main ingredient of the Yunnan Bai Yao (the white drug of Yunnan), which has, in the recent half century, won fame at home and abroad. He pointed out that it had the capacity to stop bleeding, relieve bruises, and produce analgesia. Since this drug can be taken orally or applied externally, it is extremely effective for traumatic injury and bleeding.

Besides his outstanding contribution to pharmacology, Li made useful and valid discoveries in other areas. For checking infectious diseases, the *Materia Medica* writes: "During the epidemic season, to prevent the spreading of a disease to the family, the clothes of a patient should be steamed." This was the forerunner of steam sterilization. Li also advised that ice should be applied externally to relieve high temperature and delirium, which was similar to today's practice of placing ice on a patient's forehead to subdue high fever.

Having carefully observed the animal kingdom, Li repudiated the view that fishes emerged from the seeds of weeds, and that cranes were viviparous. He asserted that they were oviparous animals. He also documented the principle that domestic feeding may change the nature of beasts. A wild animal may become tame and obey the command of his master after long-term feeding. Li gave the example of elephants that after human feeding may develop a feeling towards their feeder and render him service. Finally, the classification of the medical substances in the *Materia Medica* basically conforms to the principle that evolution proceeds in the direction of inorganic to organic, from simple to complex, from lower stratum to advanced. It was then the most advanced method of classification in the world.

The *Materia Medica* was completed in 1578. It was revised three times, then published in 1596. Incomplete statistics show that since its publication about 50 editions of it have appeared. In addition, it was translated into Japanese, English, Latin, French and German. The *Materia Medica* is not only a famous pharmaceutical book, but also contains important source material for the fields of botany, zoology and minerology. Since it also includes extensive information on chemistry, astronomy and geology, it can be said to be a 16th century Chinese encyclopedia of natural science. It is not only a precious legacy of Chinese medicine and pharmacology but also a treasure that has enriched the science of the world.

Besides *Materia Medica,* Li also wrote the *Bin Hu's Study of Pulse* and *Reference for the Eight Extraordinary Channels,* which contributed significantly to existing knowledge of the pulse and the channels. In the 1930s a German translation of the *Bin Hu's Study of Pulse* appeared.

Li lived in the middle and late stage of the decline of the feudal society when peasant revolutions took place every now and then, capitalism began to sprout in China and the ruling class pursued the so-called elixir of life. Alchemists at that time generally pandered to officials and advocated all kinds of absurdities. Faced with such idle talk, Li recommended: "One should not believe the preposterous ideas of the alchemists." To him they were extremely ridiculous, trying to do harm to people and finally harming themselves.

In short, Li Shizhen's investigation and research provide much to admire. He favoured undertaking long-term experiments and making deep observations, overcame all kinds of hardship tirelessly, opposed conservativism and dared to innovate. The contribution he made in pharmacology, medicine and other respects should be affirmed and developed.

LESSONS FROM THE ROVING DOCTORS AND *SUPPLEMENT TO MATERIA MEDICA*

"No one in the family would ever have boils if one knew groundsel." This line from a folk poem praises the effectiveness of the herb groundsel, a perennial plant belonging to the herbaceous family. In the 18th century, Zhao Xuemin, a medical expert, included that line in his *Supplement to Materia Medica.* The herb was one that Chinese people often made use of in treating boils, abscesses and skin eruptions. It can either be taken orally or applied externally. Today we know that groundsel contains ketose, which has a remarkable anti-bacteria effect.

Throughout the history of China there were numerous folk doctors who had profound clinical experience. For hundreds of years many of those doctors roved about ringing a bell through city streets and lanes, and travelled to villages to give treatment to the people, who called them "bell doctors" or "roving doctors". They especially liked to be treated by these doctors because they always used drugs that were easy to obtain. Yet in the old society these doctors were often spurned by snobbish people who thought they were not worthy of the slightest attention. Thus much of their precious experience was ignored and lost as time went by.

Zhao Xuemin, who had an innovative spirit, paid great attention to popular clinical practices and urgently felt that good remedies ought not be lost. Therefore, with the help of the folk doctor Zhao Boyun he collected and studied all the available popular clinical experience. In 1758, he wrote a book mainly distilling the experience of the roving doctors and titled it *Lessons from the Roving Doctors* because he thought that the "bell doctors" had valuable medical knowledge.

Zhao Xuemin in his *Lessons from Roving Doctors* expressed his esteem for the roving doctors because of the following three points: 1. price: one did not have to pay much for the drugs; 2. efficacy: the drugs were effective; 3. convenience: the drugs were available anywhere. He argued that one should not take their experience lightly, as "feather to the scale", asking, "who says that a feather is valueless?"

From Zhao Xuemin's great respect for the roving doctors one can tell that he was sympathetic to the working people because the roving doctors' patients were mostly the poor working masses. Zhao declared: "In drugs, it is not necessary to be expensive. Something makes a good drug if it can relieve illness as soon as it is swallowed, and if it can be found readily in hills and forests, secluded valleys or wilderness." He criticized those so-called doctors who were servile to the rich and demanded high fees. They knew how to prescribe expensive drugs and tonics but did not know how to differentiate diseases, feel the pulse or identify herbs. They were just charlatans.

Although Zhao Xuemin gave high marks to the bell roving doctors in general, he did not think all of them were praiseworthy. He charged that their ringing of the bell was only a call for attention — they were mere quacks roaming from one place to another. In the Preface to the *Lessons from the Roving Doctors* he explained that his book aimed at "helping people to shake off illness". He opposed those who used medicine as a road to wealth, a viewpoint much admired by upright people.

From childhood, Zhao Xuemin loved to read all kinds of books, especially on subjects of natural science. When he was still a lad, his father, an official, arranged for him to take the imperial examination and his brother to take up medicine. He built a villa which he called Meditation Garden and collected a fine library of medical books and planted a garden full of medicinal plants for Zhao Xuemin's brother's use in study.

But Zhao Xuemin did not follow his father's arrangement, and spent all his time studying the books in the Meditation Garden and other books. His industriousness and tireless study enabled him to achieve much in the medical field.

Constantly making notes and extracts while he was reading, after a period of time Zhao Xuemin had written "several thousand volumes" of notes. Not only did he learn from the labouring people in many respects, he also made long-term studies of herbs, how they were cultivated and their use in clinical practice. He realized more and more the truth of the saying, "The longer a thing has existed the more complicated the species will be", and therefore considered that the *Materia Medica* written by Li Shizhen was no longer satisfactory although its material was still rich. During the 100 years since its first publication, numerous new effects of many drugs had been discovered and new herbs found. Thus he determined to make a supplement and revision of the *Materia Medica*, and finally completed his *Supplement to Materia Medica*, a culmination of his 40 years of hard work and practice. From the book it can be seen that he visited more than 200 people to gather notes and material.

In writing the book, Zhao Xuemin had consulted many reference books, but he was very careful in deciding what to include in his work. He said, "Things should be listed in the book only after tests are made of their effects. . . . If anything is doubtful, put it aside rather than list it." There were many differences of opinion concerning certain herbs in the records of various books. Zhao Xuemin would cultivate such herbs in his own garden and record his own observations.

In his *Supplement to Materia Medica,* Zhao Xuemin corrected some of the errors he found in the earlier book. In the classification of the medicinal substances, he added two sorts of items: the vines and the flowers of the medicinal herbs. More than 900 kinds of medicinal substances were recorded in this book, such as *zhegucai* (Calogassa leprieurii), a treatment for ascariasis; Java brucea, used to treat amoebic dysentery; cotton seeds that suppressed pain, stopped bleeding and eliminated lice. There were also drugs introduced from abroad, like quinine for malaria and the seed of sterculia which treated hacking cough, toothache and hoarse voice.

Another valuable feature of the book was its description of the symptoms and signs of some diseases. About whooping cough, for example, Zhao Xuemin said: "Persistent coughing, in bouts, similar to asthma and yet not asthma, similar to dyspnea and yet not dyspnea. Children are usually the victims," and he added: "Often there is coughing unrelentingly in bouts more than 10 times, a stop for a while then recurrence; in severe cases, there is accompanying vomiting with pain referred to the costal region on two sides with tears and nasal discharge and generally is not relieved for several months."

Zhao Xuemin had written many books, but unfortunately the only extant ones are the *Supplement to Materia Medica* and *Lessons from the Roving Doctors.* Still, from these two books we can get an idea of the major contribution Zhao Xuemin made in the field of medicine.

"WHAT DRUGS ARE IN THE BOTTLE GOURD?"
— Forms of Chinese Drugs

"What drugs are in the bottle gourd?" This is an old common Chinese saying meaning "what has he got up his sleeve?" or, what is the hidden secret? In fact this saying relates to Chinese medicinal substances. In the *History of the Later Han Dynasty* there was a story that went as follows:

Once there was an old man who kept a medicine shop in a market place. He hung up a bottle gourd in front of the shop, and when the market closed the old man jumped into the bottle gourd and disappeared. After this story was spread around, "What drugs are in the bottle gourd?" became a common saying, and since that time hundreds of years ago, Chinese medicine shops have usually hung a bottle gourd by the door as a sign that they sell drugs. Some Chinese doctors would also hang a bottle gourd by the door as a sign for their clinical practice.

In fact, there is a still deeper relationship between the bottle gourd and Chinese medicine and pharmacology. The bottle gourd, also known as dipper squash, is itself medicine, as it may be used as a diuretic, to make edema subside. In the summer of 1973, in Hemudu, Yuyao Prefecture of Zhejiang Province, some primitive ruins were discovered. Among the excavated relics were some bottle gourd seeds, showing that at least 6,000 years ago the bottle gourd was grown in China. Now such plants are found all over the country and are used to make a common Chinese drug.

When a bottle gourd has matured, one can discard the meat and the seeds, and after the shell has dried, use it as a container. Since ancient times the Chinese people have used this gourd to contain drugs. The drug forms at that time were naturally very few and simple. In later periods, however, drugs were developed in a great variety of forms.

We know that when drugs were first used to treat diseases, people just put the drugs into the mouth raw, chewed them, then swallowed. This is the most primitive way to take medicine which is unpleasant to the taste.

Once the ancient people know how to use fire and cooked their food, the method of taking drugs was also advanced from chewing them raw to boiling them in water. Thus the decoction form was established.

According to the extant material, decoction was used as long ago as the Shang Dynasty 3,000 years ago. Yet decoction to treat diseases was undoubtedly still older than that. About 2,000 years ago, in the *Canon of Medicine*, it was mentioned that a soup of pinellia and husked sorghum was an effective remedy for insomnia. In several respects, decoction is much more advanced than chewing herbs raw. First, because the drugs were boiled it was a way of sterilizing them and making them more safe. Secondly, after the medical substances were boiled, the effective ingredients were more easily dissolved. Thirdly, boiling could attenuate the toxic side-effects of some of the drugs which might injure the stomach. Fourthly, in a decoction not just a single drug but also multiple drugs could be boiled together in a form which was easy to take and with enhanced therapeutic effect. These advantages explain why decoction is still a common method of preparing drugs in China.

After decoction came tincture, which has been discussed in the second chapter.

Next came pills. Their preparation was very crude at the

beginning. The *Canon of Medicine* already mentions the cuttle-fish-bone pill for posthemorrhage anemia and menstruation disorders. The pill was made with madder, abalone sauce, birds' eggs and cuttle-fish bone. After the Han Dynasty, the method of preparing pills improved. Honey was used to mix the ingredients, and sometimes jujube meat as well for the glutinous agent, which also gave a flavour when chewed. There were also pillets of Chinese drugs that did not require chewing before swallowing, and were convenient to preserve and transport.

Another form involves dispersion; medical substances are ground into fine or coarse powder, after which they may be taken either orally, externally, or (for some) both. One passage in the *Canon of Medicine* mentions alisma mixture for the treatment of stroke by "alcoholic wind" for internal use. The sublingual cinnamon powder described in the *Jingui Collection of Prescriptions* was put under the tongue to release its therapeutic effect. Powders in a form for external application were mostly used for direct application to the affected area or to treat skin disease. The *Jingui Collection* also mentions honey locust powder for blowing into the nose, an emergency measure to relieve syncope.

Ointment also has an ancient history, with many varieties. The *Classic of Mountains and Seas* mentions ointment made of goat fat for chapped skin. In the *Canon of Medicine*, there is pork fat which can be applied on auxiliary ulcers. A passage in the *History of the Later Han Dynasty* in the "Biography of Hua Tuo" relates that after Hua Tuo performed an abdominal operation on a patient and sutured it, he applied some "magical ointment" on the area and it healed in four or five days. The so-called "magical ointment" very possibly had the effect of suppressing pain, making inflammation subside, and promoting the healing of the trauma.

Ointment is easy to apply and transport, convenient to preserve, and inexpensive. Consequently it was very popular. After the 10th century the forms of ointments were continually increasing with the range of indications becoming wider and wider. Some of the ointments were for contusion and trauma — they stopped the pain and relieved blood stasis; some were for draining pus and reducing the inflammation of boils and abscesses; some were designed to promote the healing of a lesion and generation of new flesh and skin. Some were applied on the surface of the skin to treat internal diseases.

There was also the paste form, which could be used internally. As long ago as the Han Dynasty it was meticulously prepared in the form of an electuary: various drugs were prepared, according to the disease, then they were boiled three times; the juice was rinsed out and honey and sugar were added, after which it was boiled again until it became a thick paste which could be preserved for a long time.

Pellet originally implied that a mineral substance was extracted through heating or melting, forming a pellet. Some of the drugs very probably contained mercury, sulphur, and so on — rather violent drugs, so that generally dosages were very small. As time went by, many drugs were ground into powder and made into small pills. According to the properties of the drugs and the requirements of the treatment, the pellet might be applied externally, taken orally, or used both ways.

Drug forms had been further advanced during the Han Dynasty. The *Treatise on Febrile Diseases*, for instance, said that a mixture might become concentrated through repeated boiling. This was the beginning of "extracts". Honey might be added to improve the taste and make a decoction. This might have been the forerunner of syrup.

During the Han Dynasty, suppositories and enemas as methods to relieve constipation when it was not advisable to use purgatives were already recorded in medical literature, for instance in the *Treatise on Febrile Diseases*, which introduced the use of the anal suppository and enema. The former was called "induction by honey prescription". The method was to put honey into a bronze vessel, heat it with a low fire until it melted, then slowly mould it into the form of a stick while it was still hot. When cooled, the stick would be inserted into the rectum to help the bowels move. The earliest enema method as recorded in the *Treatise on Febrile Diseases*, was to mix the bile of a pig with a little vinegar to be infused into the rectum, causing defecation a short while later. This method was known as effective for catharsis.

There was also the fuming method introduced in the *Jingui Collection of Prescriptions* for the treatment of erosive ulcer in the rectum. First some realgar was ground into powder, put into two cylindrical tiles ignited, then directed towards the anus, where it would begin to fume.

During the Tang Dynasty, the drug form of "boiling powder" was introduced. The method was to grind the ingredients of the decoction into a fine powder. Whenever the drug was needed, the required dosage would be sectioned out and boiled; after the drugs were sieved out, it would be ready to drink. Present-day medicines in the form of powder to be mixed with water and drunk are based on the same principle.

During the Song Dynasty, patent drugs were very popular, in forms similar to those mentioned above. Tablet and syrup forms were added, as medicine and pharmacy were steadily advanced.

Since the establishment of New China, the drug forms of Chinese medicine have been building on the foundation of the past and constantly improving through research and practice. There have been many innovations in the combination and composition of drugs. Many decoction forms of the past have developed into pills, powder, syrup and capsules through extracting the effective ingredients. Especially noteworthy is the accomplishment of the injection of drugs intramuscularly and intravenously. Some synthetic forms of Western and Chinese traditional drugs were produced. Therapeutic results were enhanced. There is every reason to believe that the future will see more outstanding achievements and even more convenient drug forms.

HYGIENE AND PREVENTIVE MEDICINE IN ANCIENT CHINA

Hygiene in Chinese is "*wei sheng*", the literal translation of which is "protect life". More broadly it means keeping healthy and sanitary. This expression first appeared 2,000 years ago in the book *Zhuang Zi*.

Through the accumulation of experience in living and medical practice, the Chinese people have arrived at a knowledge of various aspects of hygiene, including diet, living habits and customs, work and rest and exercise. Equally well established are certain strategies and measures to prevent diseases.

Carved on turtle shells and ox bones in ancient China about 3,000 years ago, for example, was a word related to hygiene, the character 浴 (*yu*), meaning bath.

As early as 2,000 years ago some measures of dealing with mad dogs and prevention of rabies were recorded. *Zuoqiu Ming's Enlargement of the Spring and Autumn Annals* includes a passage reporting that in the 17th year of Duke Xiang (556 B.C.), "The people eliminated mad dogs."

The Yellow Emperor's Canon of Medicine emphasized the idea of preventive medicine, pointing out: "A wise doctor does not cure a disease, but prevents the disease. A wise statesman never brings peace to his country, but always keeps his country in peace. If the doctor waits until the disease develops to treat it or a statesman who administers his country waits until it is in turbulence it will be too late. It is equivalent to opening a well when one is thirsty or forging weapons when there is a war." In the *Canon of Medicine* a good many passages mention preventive work and early treatment.

People's emotional state is intimately related to their health and the development or modification of a disease. In the *Canon of Medicine* it says: "Anger leads to the privation of vital energy" and even caused hematemesis or diarrhea. It also says, "Joy may make one's vital energy smooth and produce good temper." It pointed out: "Uncontrolled joy or anger, or excessive cold or heat can cause unstable health."

The ancient Chinese stress on having a light heart and paying attention to preventive medicine was carried on for many generations. In the 7th century, the medical expert Sun Simiao said, "Withering in sorrow is consumptive." The 14th century famous physician Zhu Zhenheng also emphasized, "It is better to remain healthy than to receive medical treatment."

There is an old saying, "Illness enters one's body through the mouth", showing that the Chinese long ago discovered that food is an important source of diseases.

From very early times the Chinese people were concerned with water sanitation. Long ago they knew the advantages of using a well for drinking water. Water from a well is more sanitary than that from streams, lakes or ponds. The two earliest wells in China, about 4,000 years old, were discovered in Handan, Hebei Province. They were seven metres deep and two metres wide in diameter, and are dried up now.

Among the relics unearthed are many clay works of well rims or well rails. The 1972 excavation of the Han Tomb in Xincheng of Jiayuguan, Gansu Province unearthed two interesting bricks. One of them was engraved with two women carrying an urn to fetch water from a well, while the other was inscribed with the two characters meaning "drinking well water".

For maintaining the purity of water of the well, not only

would a railing be built encircling the well but also a cover. In the 11th century, the scientist Shen Kuo stated that the well should be kept covered and locked to prevent contamination of the water by insects, rats and children, and added that it was advisable to build a railing around it as well. The book *Guan Zi,* written as early as the Spring and Autumn Period, records the sanitary measure of dredging the dirt at the bottom of wells. After the Han Dynasty, a day was even fixed for clearing the well and changing the water.

The degree of purity of the water is closely related to the area where the well is situated. In the 1st century, Wang Chong in his *Discourses Weighed in the Balance* wrote: "Water in populated districts is dirty, while water in the remote areas and the wilderness is clean. The source of the water is the same but depending on the particular site, it may be filthy or pure." This shows that in early days people already knew the importance of topography for selecting one's source of water.

Food and water sanitation has a great influence on the health of the individual. *Lü's Spring and Autumn Annals,* written in the Warring States Period, states: "Anything to do with food should be clean." Wang Chong said: "Whenever a small insect falls into the wine, or when rice has been crept over by rats, it should be thrown away." Zhang Zhongjing advised that the meat of animals who died of epidemic diseases is dangerous and should not be eaten, and added: "Fruits that have dropped from the tree to the ground and bitten by ants or other insects should not be eaten."

The amount of food and water ingested was similarly recognized as critical. The *Canon of Medicine* asserts: "If one ate double the usual amount, it would damage the stomach and intestines." The 4th-century book *Bao Pu Zi* declares: "Do not eat until hungry, and do not become too full. Do not drink until thirsty, and do not drink too much." The 7th-century expert Sun Simiao said: "Do not eat and drink too much at night. . . ."

As to another aspect of hygiene, Chinese people advocated appropriate work and rest from a very early period. *Bao Pu Zi* states: "Never get up late, never oversleep," and "Don't overwork or idle the time away." Sun Simiao advised: "Irregular sleep and rest will damage the body."

The old books mention personal hygiene as well. *The Book of Rites* says: "When the cock begins to crow, get up and wash yourself," and "When the cock begins to crow, clean and sweep the rooms." The *Golden Prescriptions for Emergencies* counsels: "After you have your meal, rinse your mouth several times. This will keep your teeth healthy and your breath fresh."

In the 2nd century, in order not to let the dust spread in the air when sweeping the streets, a certain Bi Lan, according to the *History of the Later Han Dynasty*, invented a cart that could draw water, then spray it to the north and south highway while sweeping. Such equipment was in fact an urban water-spraying cart.

Through long experience the ancient people discovered that the change of weather from season to season was a hazard to health. Very often infectious disease developed during those times, so certain preventive measures were recommended. For instance, for hundreds of years, on the fifth day of the fifth moon there was a folk custom of drinking realgar wine or wine made with moxa leaves. Realgar wine would also be sprinkled on the bases of walls, or a bunch of medicinal herbs, like calamus, would be hung over the door. Some people even burned atractylodes. Realgar is now known to be effective in treating boils, abscesses and skin diseases, as it serves as a bactericide and disinfectant. Also, moxa leaves, calamus and atractylodes contain volatile oil and disinfectants. They can kill or suppress staphylococcus aureus, bacillus pyocyaneus, bacillus coli or bacillus typhi. The time around the fifth day of the fifth moon is a time for the breeding of germs, so that the above disinfectant methods are very useful.

When epidemic diseases were prevalent in ancient China, people would take preventive measures. The *Prescriptions for Emergencies* stresses that the inhabitants of a large area would not be afflicted by the disease if the members of each family took the preventive measure of the appropriate drug. Along these lines, *The Source of Diseases* (A.D. 610) explicitly advises that when one person in a family is infected very often the disease will spread, so that sometimes the whole family will die. So preventive measures are emphasized.

If an epidemic broke out, numerous people would be affected in a very short time, unless patients could be treated separately — isolated or quarantined. The *History of the Han Dynasty* records that in A.D. 2 a drought and locust disaster in many parts of the country caused many infectious diseases to spread among the people. An order from the court stipulated that inns and hostels, the temporary residences for the officials in the capital, should be used for the patients' treatment. This was the earliest government-sponsored hospitals.

By the time of the Eastern and Western Jin dynasties (265-420), the Chinese people had clearly recognized the contagious nature of leprosy, and in the Tang Dynasty a specific place was set up to treat the disease, called the "Lepers' Quarters". This was the earliest Chinese quarantine hospital.

The Chinese people realized that a healthy, well-exercised constitution and good physiological functioning could increase resistance to disease. So attention was devoted to physical training and outdoor exercises. The *Canon of Medicine* notes, for example, that some places are damp and the inhabitants exercise and labour little. So it is common for people to suffer from weakness of the extremities, muscular atrophy and motor impairment. It advises massage exercising the limbs and the joints, and deep breathing exercises with the aim of "breathing in fresh air and exhaling stale air".

During the 2nd and 3rd centuries, Hua Tuo, building on the knowledge and experience of physical training and breathing exercise inherited from the older generation, had created a set of exercises, "Five Animals Play". It imitated the gestures and the gait of the tiger, deer, bear, monkey and bird, and was designed to help build up a good constitution. He advocated that an individual, whatever his age, should continue with suitable work and exercise, which might promote digestion and absorption, blood circulation and increase resistance to disease. He compared an individual to the hinges of a door in that if it closed and opened often it would not rust. Hua Tuo's disciple Wu Pu persisted in the "Five Animals Play" exercise until the age of 90, when his eyesight, hearing ability and teeth were still good.

Shadow boxing, or Tai Ji Quan, still popular today, developed from that ancient "Five Animals Play", and is suitable for healthy persons or those with chronic disease, old and young, male or female.

The importance of taking sensible precautions against illness is stressed in *The Source of Diseases*, which gives details of how to take care of infants. It says, for instance, that they should not put on too many clothes nor should they stay inside the bed curtain or indoors all the time. If so, children are likely to become weak just as the plants in a shady place where they are protected from wind and harsh weather and would wither. It urges: "When the weather is warm and there is no wind, ask the mother to take the child out to play in the sun. More exposure to wind and sun will strengthen the body, vital energy and blood, the muscles will become firm, the child will be able to withstand wind and cold and he will be unlikely to fall ill."

In 1642, the famous doctor of infectious disease Wu Youke explained in detail in his *Epidemic Diseases* about the route of contact, features, development, prevention and treatment of infectious diseases. He emphasized that improving one's health was the best way to resist illness. These ideas further developed the viewpoint of the *Canon of Medicine* and provided more guidelines for active preventive work.

Preventive work was also reflected in maternity care. For instance, to diminish difficult labours and prevent infectious disease in the mother and newborn child, the *Golden Prescriptions for Emergencies* recommends that the maternity room should not be crowded, and should be kept quiet so that the lying-in woman can be calm rather than nervous. Two or three people staying in the room to look after her are enough. It also stresses that survivors of a death should not go into the delivery room. All these regulations are in conformity with the principle of preventing contact with infectious disease, and decreasing the possibility of complicated labour.

In the 12th century, *New Book on Child Care* stresses that in order to prevent neonatal tetanus, the scissors should be burned prior to cutting the cord; and that after cutting off the umbilical cord the incision area should always be kept dry and clean.

The ancients also came to realize that some occupations may give rise to certain diseases that can be avoided if there are appropriate preventive measures. In the 17th century a famous Chinese scientist named Song Yingxing, in his book of science and technology, the *Exploitation of the Works of Nature*, put forward a measure to prevent gas poisoning. He said that when coal is discovered, poisonous gas can make one suffocate so that before going down to the pit the miners should make a hollow bamboo pipe with one end sharpened and inserted into the coal. In that case the poisonous gas can flow out through the bamboo pipe. This might be considered as a simple labour protection measure in the old society.

As we have seen, the history of Chinese medicine furnishes abundant examples of concern with hygiene and preventive medicine. Since the founding of New China, even greater importance has been attached to preventive medicine, which has continued to progress.

TOWARDS A METHOD OF ACQUIRING IMMUNITY

— Human Vaccination

Before the invention of acquired immunity, smallpox was one of the most violent infectious diseases in the history of the world. It once seriously threatened the health of mankind and deprived thousands and thousands of people of life.

Chinese people recognized smallpox at a very early date. The previously mentioned *Handbook for Emergencies* describes it in detail, saying that smallpox appears as pustules the size of a pea all over the face and limbs, then spreads over the whole body in a very short time. The pustules will rupture from time to time and new ones will develop. The book stresses that if the disease is not treated in time, a serious case will be fatal. When cured, the face of a patient will show scars of a purplish-black colour. In a year's time the colour will gradually fade. Through their long struggle with the disease of smallpox, the Chinese people slowly mastered the preventive method called "human vaccination", which was the forerunner of acquired immunity, and an important step in the history of preventive medicine.

As far as we know, human vaccination originated in the 11th century, during the time of Emperor Zhen Zong of the Song Dynasty. There was a monk then on Mount Emei who vaccinated the son of Wang Dan, the prime minister, in order to prevent samllpox. But most researchers in Chinese medical history believe that it was in the 16th century that the Chinese people invented human vaccination, as documented in the *Medical Work of Zhang*, written by Zhang Luyu in 1695 and the *Explanation of Complete Description of Smallpox* written by Yu Maokun in 1727.

A detailed description of human vaccination methods appears in the *Golden Mirror of Medicine* of 1742, including the dry vaccine method, considered the better kind. The so-called dry vaccine involved collecting the crust of the pox of a patient who was on the road to recovery, grinding it into a fine powder and blowing it into a person's nose. This would cause a mild reaction with the effect of smallpox immunity. Another method was called the liquid vaccine method. Water would be mixed with the powder of the crust, after which some of the mixture would be swabbed into the nose cavity. These methods sometimes succeeded in preventing smallpox.

For a time after the invention of human vaccination, it was denounced by conservative people who advocated succumbing to one's divine fate. They claimed that whether anyone suffered or not was the will of god, and asked people not to believe in vaccination. Moreover, the vaccinating method was far from being perfect and the effective rate was not high. This prevented the rapid dissemination of vaccination. But subsequently some doctors improved the quality of vaccines and eventually ensured the effective rate and safety of such methods.

At the early stage of the Qing Dynasty, smallpox prevailed continuously, seriously threatening the interest and lives of the ruling class. Therefore, the imperial family and people at court were "rather enthusiastic" about receiving human vaccination. It was said that Shun Zhi, the first emperor of the Qing Dynasty, had died of smallpox; the second emperor, Kang Xi, did not catch it because he was taken care of by a nurse and lived apart from the emperor while he was suffering from the disease. Besides rushing for vaccination, the Qing government appointed a special officer to investigate smallpox incidents and quarantined those who had contracted the disease.

Human vaccination gradually attracted the attention of people from other countries, who also wanted to learn the method. According to *The Files of 1841* written by Yu Zhengxie: "In the time of Kang Xi, Russia sent people to China to study human vaccination." Emperor Kang Xi reigned from 1662 to 1722. The Russians were the earliest known students who came to China to study human vaccination.

According to *An Introduction to the History of Medicine* written by F. G. Garrison, China had adopted the method of human vaccination before Jenner invented bovine vaccination in England. The book also mentions that in March 1718 the wife of M. L. Montague, British ambassador to Turkey, had applied human vaccination to her three-year-old son, and in April 1721, she gave her five-year-old daughter another human vaccination in Britain. The method she used was probably introduced from China. Human vaccination was also introduced from China to Korea, Japan, and other Asian countries.

Although the Chinese discovery of vaccination spread to some foreign countries, and it played a role in preventing smallpox, it did not become popular, owing to its imperfection. But in the development of acquired immunization, human vaccination had undoubtedly played a pioneering role.

CHINESE HERBAL ANALEPTIC ANAESTHESIA

In Chapter 16 of the famous classical Chinese novel *Outlaws of the Marsh* is a story known as "robbing the birthday gifts by trickery". It told of an official of the Song Dynasty, Governor Liang of Daming Prefecture. Wanting to ingratiate himself with the Prime Minister Cai Jing, Liang collected from the people a treasure of pearls and jewelry worth 10,000 gold pieces. He sent 15 envoys to carry them to the Song capital (present-day Kaifeng in Henan Province) to Cai Jing's home as a birthday present.

When the peasant rebels Chao Gai and others learned about this, they thought out a plan. They would disguise themselves as pedlar selling date and wine and wait at the midpoint of the way the envoys would come, at Yellow Earth Ridge.

The envoys who were escorting the jewels, after starting off from Daming, felt very tired after a fortnight's journey across mountains and rivers, carrying their burden with poles on their shoulders. They arrived at Yellow Earth Ridge extremely exhausted and feeling very thirsty under the blazing sun. They decided to rest in the shade and set down their burden.

After a while, several pedlars came carrying date and wine with poles on their shoulders. The envoys saw them and crowded around them to buy their wine. After drinking the wine the 15 men felt giddy, as if their heads were heavy and their feet floating. They could no longer support themselves but lay on the ground. They watched their boxes of jewels and treasures loaded onto the carts, seven in all, by the date and wine pedlars. They wanted to fight and retrieve the boxs but they could "neither get up, nor move, nor speak" and just let the peasant rebels Chao Gai and his comrades push the carts away.

What kind of wine was that mentioned in the story? Why was the effect so strong? The fact was that the wine was blended with a kind of narcotic similar to what is known today as anaesthetics.

We know from other sources besides this old novel that the Chinese people had an abundant knowledge of anaesthetics.

The earliest record of surgical operations under medical anaesthesia in ancient China was in "Tang Wen", a chapter in *Lie Zi.* The story goes as follows: "Hu, the Duke of Lu, and Qi Ying of Zhao were sick and consulted Bian Que. . . . Bian Que gave them 'poisonous wine'. They became intoxicated and fell into a coma for three days, during which time Bian Que opened their chests and investigated their hearts. . . . Then he gave them the 'magical drug' whereupon they became conscious again. Subsequently they were cured and said goodbye to Bian Que and went home." From this story we can see that at least 2,000 years ago the Chinese physicians knew how to use anaesthesia and analeptic drugs.

In ancient Chinese books there was a story about the famous 2nd-century physician Hua Tuo, who knew how to use oral drugs as anaesthetic for a laparotomy. Hua Tuo's biography in the *History of the Later Han Dynasty* says: "If there is a mass in the abdomen which cannot be healed with acupuncture or medicine, then open the abdomen and remove the mass once the patient has lost consciousness under anaesthesia by swallowing *mafu*-powder with wine. Then suture the wound and apply ointment to promote the healing of the wound." The *mafu*-powder referred to here was a drug used for general anaesthesia.

The *Four Thousand Years of Pharmacy*, published in the United States in the 1920s, remarks: "Some Arabian authorities mentioned a method of anaesthesia, probably introduced from China, because Hua Tuo, the Hippocrates of China, was an expert in such a method. The drugs he used were now known as aconite, datura and henbane."

In fact, the history of the invention and application of anaesthetic drugs reaches back much earlier. The stories mentioned above are only two of the examples that could be cited. An achievement like anaesthesia was not something that could be wrought overnight but required an accumulation of experience and practice from generation to generation.

The earliest extant pharmacological book, *Shen Nong's Canon of Herbs*, mentions some drugs with anaesthetic effect, such as henbane. The book says, "One would be running along the street mad if one takes an overdose of this drug" — i.e., mental confusion due to the anaesthetic effect would result. We now know that henbane contains mainly hyoscine and atropine. The former has a sedative action, suppressing pain, and a large dose would have a hypnotic effect. The book also observes that if aconite is decocted into juice, it could poison an animal to death. This is also due to the anaesthetic effect.

After the Song Dynasty, datura flower was noted in literature as a common Chinese anaesthetic drug. In the year 1146, *My Understanding of Bian Que*, written by Dou Cai, mentioned the anaesthetic effect of datura: "After taking this drug, one will sleep and not feel pain, and it will not hurt one."

In the Yuan Dynasty (1271-1368), cavaliers were engaged by the hundreds of thousands by the imperial court. Trauma and fractures always occurred in these fighters, so that traumatological, osteological and bone-setting anaesthetics were correspondingly more developed than before. The *Doctors' Effi-*

cacious Prescriptions, written by Wei Yilin in the 14th century, gives a detailed account of the oral and external use of anaesthetics. The book correctly notes that when the anaesthetics are taken orally distinctions should be made according to the patient's age, constitution, and amount of bleeding. Later, during the Ming and Qing dynasties, numerous medical reviews and essays covered Chinese anaesthetics.

Chinese medical substances included both anaesthetic drugs and analeptic drugs. This means that after anaesthetic drugs were taken by the patient an analeptic would be given to cause prompt resuscitation. The analeptics recorded in ancient medical books were mainly derived from a single source, the liquorice complex; the source next in use was the soup of black soya beans or mung beans.

The anti-toxic properties of liquorice were already mentioned in the *Shen Nong's Canon of Herbs*. Zhang Zhongjing in the *Jingui Collection of Prescriptions* introduced the recipe of oral administration of liquorice decoction to relieve the toxic effects of henbane. Sun Simiao's *Prescriptions for Emergencies* mentions for the first time using liquorice with beans to counteract the toxins of aconite and croton. Decoctions of liquorice with soybeans were recommended to counteract poisons. The mid-17th century book *Compendium of Surgery* by Qi Kun and the 18th century book *Lessons from the Roving Doctors* by Zhao Xuemin both mention prescriptions for using liquorice to relieve the effects of anaesthetics.

More recent pharmaceutical research has shown that liquorice does indeed have a detoxication effect on many substances, like cocaine hydrochloride and chloral hydrate; it also remedies tetanus, diptheria, poisoning by globefish and snake bites. This is because liquorice contains glucose aldehydic acid, glyoxal and glycyrrhizin. Together these components produce a detoxification effect.

The use of beans for detoxification also has a very long history. Since the 2nd and 3rd centuries there have been records of using bean juice and salt to relieve the toxic effects of eating the meat of animals which had been killed by poisoned arrows. The detoxification effect of mung beans was also mentioned in medical books of various periods and very widely known.

Since 1949, Chinese pharmacology has built on and developed this part of the precious legacy of traditional Chinese medicine. A new form of anaesthetic has been invented that uses datura as the main drug. In 1970, it was for the first time successfully used in a thyroidectomy operation, and since that time research has refined and improved it. Nowadays Chinese herbal anaesthetics are administered not only orally but also through enemas and injections.

Intravenous injections of herbal anaesthetics have proved specially effective. A few minutes after injection the patient becomes drowsy and then anaesthetized. He cannot be woken up even by the sound of a bell ringing in his ear, and an operation can be smoothly performed on him. He will awake in 10 minutes after being given an analeptic injection.

Besides their anaesthetic effect, Chinese anaesthetic drugs also have excitation effects on the respiratory and central nervous systems, and keep the blood pressure normal. Hence patients anaesthetized with herbal drugs maintain normal breathing and blood pressure. The drugs have anti-shock effects as well. Up till now patients of ages ranging from newborn infants to 80-year-old people have been operated on under herbal anaesthesia, with over 100 different kinds of surgery, including heart, lung, alimentary tract, replantation of severed limb, gynecology, urinary tract, and ENT operations. Moreover, in treating mental disorders, convulsions, B-type meningitis and shocks of various causes, Chinese herbal anaesthetics have been proved effective.

Clearly the anaesthetic drugs so far developed offer many advantages. They are cheap and easily available; their method of application is easy to master; long practice shows that they are safe; and rapid resuscitations are possible with no side effects. They are especially useful for rescuing critical cases.

SURGERY IN ANCIENT CHINESE MEDICINE

Like Chinese medicine, Chinese surgery has a venerable history. The characters on ancient bones and turtle shells reveal observations about diseases of bone and joints, but they do not mention a specialty of surgery. Around the time of the Zhou Dynasty, 3,000 years ago, Chinese medicine began to divide into specialities. Altogether there were four: "disease medicine" (internal medicine), "ulcers and boils" (external medicine), diet and veterinary. The ulcers and boils department included swellings, oozing ulcers, inflammation of cuts and fractures, many of which were treated by surgeons whose methods of treatment included external application, curretting pus and blood, and applying corrosive drugs to the affected area.

Other books provide more information about the development of Chinese surgery. The *Classic of Mountains and Seas* of 2,000 years ago, for example, although not a book devoted to medicine, records many conditions that were treated by surgery, such as carbuncles, furuncles, swelling, hemorrhoids, fistula, scabies and ringworm. Some of the names given there are still in use today.

The book *Zhuang Zi* of the Warring States Period contains some stories about diseases treated through surgery. One such story goes as follows: King Hui of the State of Qin was sick and gave orders that anyone who could cure his abscesses and skin disorder would be rewarded with a coach; anyone who could cure his hemorrhoids would be rewarded with five coaches. The *Canon of Medicine* contained many articles and essays on surgery.

The most ancient surgical implement was the *bian* stone mentioned in the *Canon of Medicine*. People up till that time used stone to treat diseases instead of metal instruments because metallurgy had not yet been invented. The so-called *bian* stone was originally a rock with a sharp edge or point that people found in the wild. Later they learned to sharpen such stones themselves. A *bian* stone could be used to incise the skin to excrete pus; hence the *Canon* points out: "In the eastern districts there are many cases of ulcers and abscesses which should be treated with *bian* stone."

Metallurgy was invented in the Shang Dynasty, 3,000 years ago after which time, metal instruments for medical use began to appear. Refined bronze ware came into use as family utensils. Although bronze medical implements were probably also made at that time, they have not yet been unearthed.

The methods of treating pus formation with acupuncture mentioned in the *Canon* are basically correct. In addition, the section on carbuncles and furuncles says that when flesh decays it will become putrid and if the pus is not removed the bone and marrow will be affected. It points out that if acupuncture is used to treat abscesses, the needle has to be inserted into the soft, putrid area in order to investigate the size and depth of the abscess. Then the needle will puncture it to the required depth. This method does actually help discharge pus.

Thromboangiitis often starts with pain in the toes; gradually the toes become discoloured and necrosis develops. The condition is rather difficult to treat, and if the necrosis area is large and the pain and infection beyond control, modern medicine employs amputation. The *Canon* of 2,000 years ago describes this disease correctly — then it was known as "gangrene". It says that it occurs primarily in the toes, and if blackish decolouration is present it is incurable, but if decolouration is absent it will not be fatal. It recommends that if the illness continues to develop the toes should be amputated to save the patient's life.

We know now that thromboangiitis is caused by a pathological change in vascular membranes. Gradually an embolus develops, pain is present, and local tissue becomes discoloured and necrotic. Western medicine did not recognize thromboagiitis until Von Winiwarter, a German, and Leo Buerger, an American, gave detailed reports of the disease in 1878 and 1908, respectively.

The *Canon of Medicine* also gives detailed descriptions of diseases of traumatology and osteology, noting that if one falls from a high place, there will be blood stagnation, abdominal distention, retention of urine and stool, and paralysis.

At present transplantation of internal organs, particularly hearts and kidneys, is possible when an organ has lost its function. Two thousand years ago in China there was a story about the transplantation of internal organs. The chapter "Tang Wen" in *Lie Zi* tells a story about Bian Que performing an operation of transplanting a patient's heart after given him an anaesthetic drug. Of course the scientific level of those days would not allow heart transplantations but such daring speculations of that day are significant.

Chunyu Yi, a doctor who was the earliest to keep case histories in China, was born around the 2nd century. He had once worked in a storehouse, so that people used to call him the "store master" or Cang Gong. The chapter "Bian Que and Cang Gong" in the *Records of the Historian* tells of 25 cases handled by Chunyu Yi, one of which was a tale of lumbovertebral trauma, as follows: One day Dr. Chunyu attended a banquet to which he had been invited. When the guests were seated he noticed that the gestures and appearance of the host's brother-in-law were somewhat abnormal. He said: "Four or five days ago, something must have happened to your lumbar and costal region. You cannot straighten your back, nor can you bend down, and at the same time you must have difficulty in urination. . . ." The host's brother-in-law replied: "It is true that I have a lumbovertebral disorder. Four or five days ago it was rainy, and several sons-in-law of my sister's came to my home to visit. They played with my large square stones and tried to lift it up. I wanted to try, yet no matter how hard I tried, I could not lift it, so I put it down again. At night, I felt pain in my back and then I had difficulty in urination. I do not feel any better even today." Chunyu Yi diagnosed that he had sprained his lower back during his attempt to lift the stone. He prescribed some pills for him to relax the tendons and promote blood circulation. After 18 days of treatment the host's brother-in-law recovered.

What kind of drugs Chunyu Yi used we do not know. Unfortunately that was not recorded. But in *Shen Nong's Canon of Herbs*, compiled around the same time, there are records of such drugs to treat traumatic injury and bone fractures as glutinous rehmannia, teasel root and garden burnet.

During the Three Kingdoms period, Chinese surgery succeeded in performing a laparotomy under general anaesthesia. The doctor who performed the operation was none other than the famous Hua Tuo. Hua Tuo (around 145-208) was a folk doctor with ample experience. He practised medicine in the region where Anhui, Jiangsu, Shandong and Henan provinces join. By his day, iron casting and steel tempering had developed, forging some high quality knives and needles which fostered the development of surgery. According to the biography of Hua Tuo in the *History of the Later Han Dynasty*, he once applied general anaesthesia to perform a laparotomy on a patient, removing a tumour from the intestine or stomach. Thus surgery had reached a very high level at that time.

Some of the diseases treated through surgery were also treated with oral administration of drugs. The well-known doctor Zhang Zhongjing, a little later than Hua Tuo, described in his medical works his experience of treating intestinal obstructions and appendicitis with herbal drugs.

Around the 5th century, in the Jin Dynasty, one great innovation was orthopedic operations. The *History of the Jin Dynasty* told a story of the repairing of a harelip. It said: "The doctor 'cut and repaired' it for a man who had congenital harelip. He regained his normal look."

Around this period appeared the *Ghosts' Prescriptions of Liu Juanzi* compiled by Gong Qingxuan, which presents Liu Juanzi's experiences of treating traumatic injury and infection during the time he was with the army. The book introduces techniques to incise abscesses and drain pus. When operating on a boil, it recommends, the base should be cut to help the pus flow out. For a deep-rooted carbuncle, it stresses using red, hot needles to puncture and drain off the pus. This was a significant measure in preventing the spread of inflammation.

In the Sui and Tang dynasties (581-907 A.D.), Chinese surgery developed further. In 601, *The Source of Diseases* compiled by Chao Yuanfang and others, saw publication. This is the earliest extant book concerning etiology and pathology, and includes much about diseases which can be treated by surgery.

For example, in the book is the earliest record of intestinal diseases and intestinal anastomosis operations. It say that if the reticular membrane drops out from an abdominal wound, it can be removed after binding it with silk thread. If there is inflammation in the wound, suture is not desirable because it is necessary to drain the pus. Another point stressed in the book is that if any fragments of bone, thorns or any foreign body are lodged in the wound after a fracture, it has to be cleared first, or else it will become putrid and the wound will be long in healing. It also describes the sequela of local paralysis and numbness after an injury to the nerves and blood vessels, and gives an illustration of an open fracture complicated by tetanus, with symptoms and signs correctly featured.

In 624, there was a department of boils and abscesses and a massage section in the Imperial Medical Academy established by the Tang government which also treated external disorders such as falls and contusion. This gives us an idea of the development of Chinese surgery at that time.

In the 7th century the famous doctor Sun Simiao gave a further account of the treatment and prevention of abscesses. He pointed out: "When examining an abscess with the finger, if it rises and falls with the finger, the abscess has matured (pus has formed) and surgery should be applied in time to drain off the pus." He also correctly observed that an abscess was liable to be a complicated matter if a patient had diabetes; one had to be especially careful to prevent such an occurrence.

The mid-9th century *Secret Prescriptions for the Treatment of Fracture and Reunion* by Lin Daoren is the earliest extant book on osteology. It explains that fractures should be correctly repositioned, medicine applied and then the bones set with splints. But if a fracture is accompanied by muscular injury and bleeding, onion juice or medicated soup should be boiled to bathe and cleanse the wound before reducing to fractured part and applying medicine. Then silk or soft paper should be spread over the wound, splints placed around it and the whole thing tied with bandages; the dressing should be cleaned over two or three days, washed with onion water if necessary. The book emphasizes that after the joints are reset, "move them often", which would promote early recovery of their function and prevent or diminish deformation. These measures are of significant value. Another recommendation of the book that still applies to today's surgery is the "sharp knife" method to expand the wound, clear off dead tissue and drain off the pus.

During the Song Dynasty, surgery, traumatology and osteology steadily improved. The famous 12th century painting, *Riverside Scene at Qingming Festival* by Zhang Zeduan depicts a city scene in which one building bears the sign, "Clinic for Treating Traumatic Injury". Hence we know that treatment of bone injuries had advanced by that time.

From the years 1111-1117 we have the book *General Records of Effective Cures,* in which Chinese medical literature prior to the Song Dynasty is collected. Prescriptions for simple and efficacious drugs from the people are gathered and arranged. For diseases usually treated by surgery, the book advocates both oral administration and external application of drugs. Arsenic was then used to treat hemorrhoids, for example, a forerunner of the present method for "necrosis of the hemorrhoids".

The Yuan Dynasty saw the appearance of the *Doctors' Efficacious Prescriptions,* compiled by Wei Yilin, an important book on surgery and bone fractures. It was based on ancient knowledge as well as his own experience in treatment. Published in 1345, the book concentrates on surgical diseases, the dislocation of joints and bone fractures. It describes methods for repositioning dislocated shoulders, elbows, knees and ankle joints, and advises that after repositioning, the joints have to be flexed and extended appropriately, taking care to prevent redislocation. As for splintered fractures, it stresses that before surgery a dose of oral anaesthetic should be given to the patient.

Surgery continued to develop in the Ming Dynasty. In 1531 the *Surgery Cases* by Wang Ji was published, in which he claimed that the body as a whole should be taken into account when giving surgical treatment. He wrote: "When treating external diseases the internal condition should also be considered; consideration of internal conditions is necessary for the treatment of external disorders." He pointed out that if treatment considered only the superficial disorders and neglected to regulate the internal portion of the body, it could be compared with "discarding the origin to chase after the floating shadow."

In 1617 there was the *Orthodox Manual of Surgery* by Chen Shigong, an important surgical work of the Ming Dynasty. The author stressed that both internal and external treatment should be judiciously considered. He opposed the indiscriminate use of surgery, but advocated that when surgery was necessary it should be done early. He introduced a technique for suturing the trachea to rescue a patient who attempted suicide by slitting his throat. He said: "If there is still breathing and the body is not yet cold, then suture up the incision immediately with silk thread." In the book he detailed both successful and unsuccessful cases.

The *Brief Medical Cases* by Sun Zhihong in 1629 recounts a method of treating a congenital occlusion of the anus. He wrote: "It is rare to find a newborn infant without an anus, and it will die in 10 days if defecation is impossible. It is necessary to perforate the anus at once with a fine knife, first making an aperture, then rolling silk as thick as a small finger, soaking it in sesame oil and inserting it into the aperture. The anus will not close again."

The Qing government ordered the publication of the *Golden Mirror of Medicine* in 1724, which not only contains much information on surgery and osteology, it also illustrates the surgical implements of the day. It mentions the "lumbar pop" which can treat misplacement of the lumbar vertebra, equalling the effect of today's lumbosacral supporters for lower back pain. The *Golden Mirror* introduces the technique of "fixture" for treating fractures of the spinal column, equivalent in effect to a splint or a back supporter of today for treatment of a vertebral fracture. There is also the so-called "bamboo screen" to remedy a fracture of the upper or lower limbs — equivalent to the plaster fixation of modern medicine, only with the advantage of "combining fixation and ability to move", so that the limb would better recover its function.

Another development occurred in 1840, with the publication of the *Prescriptions for Traumatology*, written by Jiang Kaoqing. He mentioned using grafting to treat a splintered fracture which was a new way of handling bone injuries.

To sum up, the great accomplishments of early Chinese surgery were followed by medical stagnation in feudal times. Chinese surgery did not develop then as it should have, owing to the restrictive feudal codes. Later, Chinese surgery was hindered by its lack of attention to scientific knowledge. In New China the medical personnel trained in traditional and Western medicine are encouraged to learn from each other, absorbing each others' strong points so as to better serve the sick and wounded and keep its people healthy.

CHINESE MEDICINE'S UNIQUE THERAPY

— Acupuncture and Moxibustion

Acupuncture and moxibustion therapy form a distinctive part of Chinese medicine, with a venerable history. They are also popular treatments because they are easily applied, the range of indications is broad, the effect is fast, and they are safe and economical. For the past several thousand years, acupuncture and moxibustion have not only played an important role in preserving the health of the Chinese people, but they also spread abroad early on. More and more people have become convinced of their therapeutic value.

Acupuncture and moxibustion are two different kinds of therapeutic methods but they both treat conditions by selecting points according to the theory of the channels. They are similar and are always considered side by side. The *Canon of Medicine* says in one of its passages, for example, "If it is not suitable to apply acupuncture, apply moxibustion".

According to the record of ancient Chinese medical books, acupuncture needles were at first made not of metal but of sharp little flat stones — *bian* stone, they called it. Xu Shen (58-147) in his *Analytical Dictionary of Characters* explained, "*Bian* means to treat disease by pricking with a stone." In other words, a small sharp stone was used to prick or press on a certain area of the body surface to treat diseases. This makes *bian* stone the most primitive acupuncture implement for therapeutic purposes. Later on, when people sharpened stones to make needles they sharpened bones and bamboo for that purpose also. After pottery was invented people also sometimes treated diseases with "pottery needles" — that is to say, sharp fragments of pottery pricked superficially at a certain point on the body. Following the invention of metallurgy there were bronze, iron and silver needles as well. Nowadays stainless steel needles, much more refined and convenient, are used.

The invention of metallurgy not only provided the basic material for making metal needles but also the possibility of making needles in various shapes for different purposes. The *Canon of Medicine* recorded the ancient "nine kinds of needles", their shapes, length and usage. These are as follows:

1. Arrowhead needle. The head is shaped like an arrow, very large and sharp. Suitable for superficial pricking.
2. The round needle. The body is like a column, the head round like an egg. Mainly for massaging at the points.
3. The blunt needle. The head is blunt, with a thick body. Mainly for pressing.
4. The three-edge needle. The body is round, with a triangular, sharp head. Used to cause bleeding.
5. Sword needle. It has cutting edges on both sides like a sword. Used to make incisions to drain pus.
6. Round sharp needle. The body is thick, the head is round and sharp. Used for fast pricking.
7. The filiform needle. The body is thin as hair. Extensively used.
8. The long needle. It is as long as 20 cm. and the longest needle of all. Used for puncturing an area with thick muscle.
9. The large needle. The body is thick and the head is round. Used for treating the joints.

The introduction of the nine kinds of needles increased the methods of acupuncture, enhanced its therapeutic effect, and enlarged its range of indications. Thus their appearance is a landmark in the development of acupuncture. The oldest metal acupuncture needles were unearthed in 1968, in the tomb of Prince Liu Sheng of Zhongshan and his wife from the time of the Western Han Dynasty (206 B.C.-A.D. 24) in Mancheng, Hebei Province. In the tomb were also discovered four golden needles still in perfect condition and five broken silver ones. The discovery corroborated ideas of the long history of Chinese acupuncture therapy.

Moxibustion, the other distinctive form of Chinese therapy, was discovered in ancient times when people would sit around a fire to keep warm. They found that heat was able to relieve certain pains in their bodies. Perhaps also while using fire they inadvertently found that a burn could unexpectedly ameliorate certain symptoms of their disease. Thus moxibustion was developed. Ancient books found in 1973 in Changsha, in the third Han tomb of Mawangdui, mention moxibustion and the channels, but not acupuncture.

They did not use moxa leaves (*Artemisia chinensis*) at the beginning but various things, such as branches and grass. Later on they used charcoal and bamboo sticks and finally moxa leaves, sulphur, realgar and rush, though the primary substance used was moxa leaves.

Through long years of practice, ancient people understood the advantages of moxa leaves, including the fact that moxa leaves that had been kept for several years yielded better therapeutic results than ones that were newly collected. In *Mencius* of the Warring States Period there is a passage, "Search out moxa leaves that have been kept for three years to treat the disease that has lingered for seven years." Thus we can see that moxibustion was widely used to treat diseases at least as early as 2,000 years ago.

Aged moxa leaves are better for moxibustion because the

fire burns more evenly and mildly and the heat gives one the sensation of deep muscle penetration. Their effect was introduced in ancient Chinese medical literature. Li Shizhen in his *Materia Medica* said that "*Artemisia chinensis* (moxa) had the effect of warming the spleen and stomach and dispelling cold and damp". The Chinese people knew very early that the smoke of burning moxa leaves could drive mosquitoes away. Now experiments have shown that moxa leaves contain volatile oil which to a certain extent is bacteriostatic. Thus we can understand the advantages of treating diseases through fuming moxa leaves.

Throughout *The Yellow Emperor's Canon of Medicine* are numerous discussions of acupuncture and moxibustion. One part, "Ling Shu", describes in detail the theory of the channels and points, the equipment and methods of needling, and its indications and contraindications. This part of the book was later called the *Canon of Acupuncture* because it lays the foundation for the therapy.

Experience had taught that if certain points were punctured, a sensation of soreness, tingling, distention and heaviness would appear, and such sensation would travel along a definite line. When they realized that many points had the same or similar effects, they joined the points together, forming lines. Thus the concept of channels was born. At the same time, they discovered that puncturing or performing moxibustion on one point or points might treat a disease in some other part of the body or an internal organ. They then deduced that the channels established a special relation between certain superficial part of the body and other parts of the body, and between the internal organs and the body surface. Thus "Ling Shu" said: "Internally, channels relate to the viscera and externally, they link with the limbs and joints".

The ancients called the "line" that runs longitudinally a

"channel" (*jing*), or route, and large and small branches that diverge "collaterals" (*luo*), i.e., nets. According to the channel theory, these channels and collaterals running longitudinally and latitudinally through the body, internally and externally, make one integral "channel system". The channels are also held to govern the adjustment and maintenance of various functions of the human body.

Of the therapeutic effects of acupuncture and moxibustion mentioned in *Canon of Medicine,* the outstanding one is the suppression of pain. It says: "As soon as the needle has reached the point the pain stops at once." The chapter on "The Tendon" in "Ling Shu" emphasizes many times, "Where there is pain there is a point." Thus therapists were directed to select points from the area where the pain was.

A Classic of Acupuncture and Moxibustion, written by Huangfu Mi (215-282), is the oldest extant book devoted exclusively to acupuncture and moxibustion. Originally Huangfu was not a physician, but because he was afflicted with rheumatoid arthritis when he was middle-aged, he took up the study of medicine, especially acupuncture. He summarized the accomplishments of his predecessors and systematized all the material on acupuncture scattered throughout the *Canon of Medicine.* In addition, combining his own wisdom and experience with the material in *Mingtang Points for Acupuncture Treatment,* particularly its descriptions of the points of the head, face, chest, abdomen and back, its methods of treating all kinds of diseases, he wrote *A Classic of Acupuncture and Moxibustion.* This book records 649 points and discusses the theory of acupuncture and moxibustion, manipulation methods, indications and contraindications. This book was very influential to later generations, both in China and abroad.

During the Tang Dynasty, there were two outstanding developments in acupuncture: First, colourful charts with illustrations of channels and points appeared, and secondly, acupuncture and moxibustion became independent academic courses of study.

The Tang Dynasty book *Golden Prescriptions for Emergencies* includes coloured charts of the channels and points, of which the book says: "The 12 channels are painted in five colours, the eight extraordinary channels painted in green." Actually, long before the appearance of this book acupuncture charts had been drawn up, but they were not in colour. Furthermore, since they required numerous times of tracing and drawing, mistakes had crept in. Thus Sun Simiao, using charts made by the famous doctor Zhen Quan and others as the foundation, made coloured acupunctural charts from the 6th century to the middle of the 7th century, but unfortunately these have been lost.

In the *Old History of the Tang Dynasty* was a biography of Zhen Quan which included a story about his treatment with acupuncture: A certain archer named Ku Diyu could not draw the bow to shoot the arrow because of pain around his shoulder. He had seen many doctors but to no avail. When he consulted Zhen Quan, however, the latter told him that one sitting of acupuncture would cure him. He asked the patient to take the bow and arrow in hand and face the target. Then he punctured at the point "Jian Yu".[1] When the patient then drew the bow, the arrow flew and hit the target without difficulty.

Acupuncture became an independent academic specialty in the Tang Dynasty, as we know from accunts of the departments of the Imperial Medical Academy at that time. Acupuncture

---

[1] At the anterior and inferior border of the acromio-clavicular joint, below the acrominon when the arm is in full abduction. Indications are pain and impairment of movement of the elbow and arm, disorders of the shoulder joint and its surrounding soft tissue, or numbness in the upper limb.

professors, instructors, assistants and technicians were assigned to the acupuncture department to be responsible for teaching and treatment. Students specializing in acupuncture were enrolled every year.

Three important developments in acupuncture occurred in the Song Dynasty. First, there appeared in 1026 a national acupuncture book *New Illustrated Manual on the Points for Acupuncture and Moxibustion on the Bronze Figure* written by Wang Weiyi, a renowned doctor, who arranged all the acupuncture material available from the past. After thorough textual research he verified the names of 354 points and the locations of 657 points. He also described the depth for puncture of each point, the effects of acupuncture and many other relevant findings.

Secondly, while writing the book Wang Weiyi had two acupuncture models cast. Thus in 1027 there appeared two life-sized bronze acupuncture figures. On the surface were points with their names indicated. This helped to standardize reference to the acupuncture points.

Thirdly, not long after the *New Illustrated Manual* was published, its contents were engraved on two stone tablets more than two metres high and seven metres wide, which were erected in the Song capital Bianliang (now Kaifeng, Henan Province) so that those who were studying acupuncture could trace them.

Acupuncture and moxibustion were very popular in the Song Dynasty because the ruling class advocated the therapeutic methods besides receiving treatment themselves. According to the *History of the Song Dynasty*, in the first year of the Jingyou period (1034), Emperor Ren Zhong was sick; the imperial doctors treated him with medicine but without success. Before long, someone recommended a doctor named Xu Xi, who after examining the patient predicted: "He can be cured if acupuncture is done below the heart between the collaterals." People in the emperor's court who heard this thought it would be too dangerous, and refused to let Xu Xi puncture. First they and the enunchs tested it on their own bodies and reported "no harm done", so that the emperor received acupuncture and recovered in no time.

After Xu Xi cured the Song emperor, he was appointed medical officer of the Imperial Medical Academy and rewarded with precious gifts. Xu Xi asked if he could use his gifts to build a temple for Bian Que whom he thought had contributed much to medicine. The court agreed, and in the west corner of the capital the Temple of Bian Que was erected.

During the 1260s, Kublai Khan ruled the north part of China. The two bronze acupuncture figures were moved to Yanjing (Beijing) and had them repaired because their surfaces were blurred. Not until the Ming Dynasty, in 1443, were new bronze acupuncture figures cast.

Two celebrated acupuncturists in the Ming Dynasty were Gao Wu and Yang Jizhou. In 1537 Gao Wu compiled and wrote *Eminent Acupuncture,* which includes information on channels, points, treatment, selection of points for different diseases and manipulation, as well as his own ideas. Prior to compiling this book he had collected all the important acupuncture works like *Canon of Medicine* and summarized them in *Essentials of Acupuncture and Moxibustion,* for the use of beginners.

Since Gao Wu believed that numerous mistakes in the location of points had arisen after the Song Dynasty, and that there were differences in the location of points in men, women and children, in the mid-16th century he cast three figures of a man, woman and child to show the respective location of points.

At the end of the 16th century, Yang Jizhou collected and

abstracted the acupuncture works of past centuries and combining their information with his own experience he wrote the *Compendium of Acupuncture and Moxibustion*. He included important records with annotations. He also discussed the channels and points, manipulation, indications and cases, and told of his experience in combining medicine and acupuncture. Especially valuable for present-day researchers are his extensive quotations from ancient medical sources, some of which were later lost. Published in 1601, the *Compendium of Acupuncture and Moxibustion* has become well known abroad and in China.

Before the 18th century the Qing Dynasty respected acupuncture. In 1742, by order of the court, the physician Wu Qian and others completed a series of works the *Golden Mirror of Medicine* and in the year 1744 the court awarded each of the editors a copy of the book and manikin showing acupuncture points and channels. But after the 19th century the Qing government turned about and arbitrarily trampled upon acupuncture, which they said "is not the way to serve the upper classes". In 1822 they banned acupuncture altogether. By the end of the Qing Dynasty they even cancelled the subject of acupuncture in the royal medical examinations for the Imperial Medical Academy.

During the period of Koumintang rule, the development of acupuncture encountered a still greater obstacle when the government tried to ban traditional Chinese medicine. Yet because acupuncture suited the people's need in medical care, it kept on spreading extensively among the people.

After the birth of New China, acupuncture developed quickly. Ancient medical books were republished and many new ones appeared. Research institutes of acupuncture were built in various places and departments of it established in traditional Chinese medical colleges or at least acupuncture courses included in the curriculum. Medical personnel and scientific workers began to apply modern scientific methods to systematize and develop acupuncture. In recent years they have created innovative therapeutic methods such as finger, ear, nose, face, scalp, fire, electron, water, wrist and ankle needles.

Acupuncture anaesthesia is an outstanding case in point. In 1958 Chinese doctors who knew on the basis of their experience that some points could suppress pain began to use acupuncture to treat patients who suffered pain after an operation. They met with success. They therefore predicted that acupuncture could be used as anaesthesia. After further experiments they tried it with tonsillectomy. Later, many clinics and hospitals used it for tooth extractions, thyroidectomy and hernia repair; they also were successful.

After 1959 acupuncture anaesthesia was applied in operations of the thorax, limbs and abdomen, removal of a tumour from the brain, a heart surgery operation under extracorporeal cardio-pulmonary circulation — many operations big and small. Acupuncture anaesthesia has many advantages: it is simple and secure to use, easy to popularize, reduces the suppression of physiological functions, has a wide range of indications and allows an early post-operative recovery without side effects. Some patients who cannot tolerate drug anaesthesia for one reason or another are able to have surgery with acupuncture anaesthesia.

In 1971 the *People's Daily* reported the invention of acupuncture anaesthesia and drew the attention of domestic and foreign medical circles. Since 1975, acupuncture classes for foreign doctors, warmly supported by the World Health Organization and many countries, have been established in Beijing, Shanghai, Nanjing and other cities. In December 1979, WHO made a decision to apply acupuncture in the treatment of 43 kinds of diseases, including periodic attacks of migraine, constipations, colds and cataract.

The success of acupuncture anaesthesia has not only enriched the field of acupuncture, but also posed new problems of research for the attention of scientists in medicine and other fields. With acupuncture anaesthesia some hospitals have been able to ban the old regulation of "fasting" and the insertion of the stomach tube. After an operation, the patient can eat and move around, which accelerates recovery.

Up to now, acupuncture, moxibustion and acu-anaesthesia have attained a high level of accomplishment. But there is still no satisfactory scientific explanation of the points and channels and the reasons these methods can treat disease or anaesthetize. Moreover, when using acupuncture anaesthesia to operate there are still problems, such as the subtotal suppression of pain, muscular tension and reactions from traction of the viscera. There is still room for further advancement and deeper research in the area of acupuncture and moxibustion.

ANCIENT PHYSICIANS' CONCEPT OF TUMOURS

Tumours and cancers are not recent phenomena in the medical history of China, but quite ancient ones, as we know by looking at China's oldest medical books. The word "tumour" can be found in the *Canon of Medicine* of 2,000 years ago, which lists tumours of different areas of the body such as tendon tumour, intestinal tumour, and so on. Other books mention benign and malignant tumours, often by different names. Many of the ancient medical books discuss tumour pathology. Although some of the discussions offer only conjectures, there are many reasonable explanations.

According to Chinese medicine, *qi*, or the vital energy, and blood are the basis of the proper functioning of the entire body. *Qi* means not only the air of the atmosphere but also the minute nutritional essence that circulates inside the body and the functional activity of the viscera. Many factors both outside and inside the body can make the *qi* and blood abnormal, in which case the so-called *qi* stagnation or blood stasis is caused and diseases occur. According to Chinese medicine, the causes of tumours include excessive tension, external disease factors, senility, or the changing of food and habits which lead to *qi* stagnation and blood stasis. Also any abnormal material obstruction produced in the body, or dysfuntion or derangement of the viscera and so on could cause tumours.

A malignant tumour in Chinese medicine is called "*ai*" — literally, "rock". Why? Inspection usually reveals that a cancer is hard and fixed, with an uneven surface, just like rock.

In the extant Chinese medical literature, the disease of cancer was discussed long ago, in the 12th-century *Precious Book for Prescriptions,* for instance, and the *Renzhai Guide to Diagnosis and Prescriptions* of 1264. The latter gives the earliest and most concise Chinese description of cancer, saying that the upper part is high and the lower part deep like a rock cave, that it spreads in branches, that its poisonous root keeps reaching more and more deeply, and that once it takes root it will eventually reach the interior. In the male it develops mostly in the abdomen, while in the female it develops mostly in the breast, neck, back or arm.

There are many other descriptions of the main symptoms, signs and characteristics of cancer in the Chinese medical literature of various generations, many of which are essentially correct. *The Source of Diseases* records, ". . . sudden swelling of the flesh and skin, at the beginning as big as a plum and gradually developing without pain or pruritus — this is called a tumour."

A more specific description was given of lip cancer. The ancient Chinese medical literature says it is like a cocoon. The *Orthodox Manual of Surgery* of Chen Shigong published in 1617 also gives an illustration. It says that at the beginning there is a lump as big as a bean on the lip, then it gradually grows to the size of a silk cocoon. It is very hard and painful, and indicates an incurable disease. Lip cancer, the book says, may be due to general factors of deep sorrow, or irascibility, or to local factors like irritating the lip by taking fried, crispy or roasted food. Modern medicine holds that smoking a pipe for a long period of time may cause lip cancer because it irritates the lips.

In Chinese medicine, esophagus cancer includes difficulty in swallowing due to problems in the throat, esophagus and stomach. *Canon of Medicine* says that obstruction of the esophagus (in most cases, cancer) is due to over-anxiety. That is to say, emotion is the inducing factor. In Chinese medicine there is also a disease called "regurgitation". In the early 3rd century, Zhang Zhongjing described it thus: "The food that had been taken in the morning would be vomited out in the evening and the food that had been taken in the evening would be vomited out the next morning". The cause of such disease is mainly obstruction in the stomach or intestine due to ulcer or cancer.

The numerous descriptions of breast cancer include one in the *Orthodox Manual of Surgery*. It says that at the beginning it is as big as a bean. It may be without pain or pruritus for the first two or three years. Then it becomes gradually bigger and constantly painful. It will develop like two or three chestnuts heaped together. The local area will gradually change colour, and become ulcerated and fetid. The concave part is like a rock cave, the convex part like lotus seeds. Later, it is very painful, like drilling to the heart. The patient will feel exhausted and the disease is considered incurable.

Breast cancer mostly develops in women, very seldom in men. *Standard Treatments in Diseases* published in 1608 by Wang Kengtang, however, records a case of breast cancer in a male. It says that this man had taken the official examination several times, failed each time, and as a result was very depressed. Then the nipple of his left breast began to exude a small quantity of fluid. Before long masses appeared beside the nipple and grew, becoming ulcerated and cave-like. Because of a delay in diagnosis and proper treatment, it was incurable. This description is in conformity with what we now know of the development of breast cancer.

As for abdominal tumours, the *General Records of Effective*

Cures, published around 1111-1117, says in a description of a patient that he had a mass like a cup in his abdomen that was fixed and could not be pushed. Doctors were consulted but of no avail. Finally the abdomen became swollen, the body emaciated and he died. Undoubtedly the man was suffering from abdominal cancer.

In Chinese medicine, cancer is sometimes called "lost-of-lustre". Why? Gao Bingjun's *Comprehension of Ulcers*, published in the year 1805, says it is because at the final stage of the disease the patient often loses all his lustre just like a withering tree with its bark and branches all dry up. The book also says that such diseases usually start anterior or posterior to the ear or in the neck. At the beginning it is as big as a chestnut, fixed and hard as stone. At the first stage there is no heat or cold, then afterwards pain appears and it ulcerates; fluid and blood will ooze out and it will have a surface like an uneven rock. It also says such a disease, like breast cancer, is always a pernicious disease. This description seems to include thyroid carcinoma and cancers that have spread from the lymph nodes of the neck.

Although doctors of Chinese medicine in the past recognized that some of the tumours were incurable, they did not fear their fierceness. At first they treated the body as a whole and reinforced the general health, then they administered medicines directed to the tumour and operated if they thought it necessary.

The "Plain Question" in *Canon of Medicine* mentions tumours, and says that the method of treating them is to make them subside.

The earliest recorded surgical removal of a tumour was in the 3rd century. In the "Records of Emperor Jing Di" in the *History of the Jin Dynasty* it is said that "at first, the emperor got a tumour in his eye and he commanded an operation to be performed."

The *Elementary Medicine* published by Li Yan in 1575 mentions using a very sharp knife to remove an adipose tumour. It also describes the method of treating some tumours that have grown as big as an eggplant, which is to apply medicinal corrosion to the base of the tumour and let it disappear by itself.

As for treating tumours with medicines, doctors of Chinese medicine adopt the principle of differentiating a syndrome according to the individual condition. On the one hand it had to strengthen the patient's body resistance so as to let him have the power to expel the disease, and on the other hand the doctors have to consider the treatment to be directed to the tumour. This could only be done by considering each case individually.

After the birth of New China, Chinese medicine made some progress and amassed new experience in preventing and treating tumours. By integrating Chinese and Western medicine and using modern scientific knowledge, more effective methods to prevent and treat tumours will undoubtedly be discovered in future years.

BIBLIOGRAPHY

Analytical Dictionary of Characters
说文解字

Bao Pu Zi
抱朴子

Bin Hu's Study of Pulse
濒湖脉学

Book of Rites, The
礼记

Book of Songs
诗经

Book of the Prince of Huainan, The
淮南子

Brief Medical Cases
简明医彀

Canon of Acupuncture and Moxibustion
针灸甲乙经

Canon of Herbs with Annotations
本草经集注

Categories of Prescriptions
医方类聚

Classic of Acupuncture and Moxibustion, A
针灸甲乙经

Classic of Mountains and Seas
山海经

Classic on Pulse
脉经

Compendium of Acupuncture and Moxibustion
针灸大成

Compendium of Materia Medica
本草纲目

Compendium of Surgery
外科大成

Comprehension of Ulcers
疡科心得集

Discourses Weighed in the Balance
论衡

Doctors' Efficacious Prescriptions
世医得效方

Elementary Medicine
医学入门

Eminent Acupuncture
针灸聚英

Engishiki
延喜式

Epidemic Diseases
温疫论

Essentials of Acupuncture and Moxibustion
针灸节要

Explanation of Complete Description of Smallpox
痘科全镜赋集解

Exploitation of the Works of Nature
天工开物

Files of 1841, The
癸巳存稿

Four Thousand Years of Pharmacy

General Records of Effective Cures
圣济总录

Ghosts' Prescriptions of Liu Juanzi
刘涓子鬼遗方

Golden Mirror of Medicine
医宗金鉴

Golden Prescriptions for Emergencies
备急千金要方

Guan Zi
管子

Handbook for Emergencies
肘后备急方

History of the Han Dynasty
汉书

History of the Jin Dynasty
晋书

History of the Later Han Dynasty
后汉书

History of the Song Dynasty
宋史

History of Three Emperors
史记补三皇纪

Important Golden Prescriptions
千金宝要方

Introduction to the History of Medicine, An
F. G. Garrison

Jingui Collection of Prescriptions
金匮要略方论

Lessons from the Roving Doctors
串雅

Lie Zi
列子

Lü's Spring and Autumn Annals
吕氏春秋

Medical Work of Zhang
张氏医通

Mencius
孟子

Mingtang Points for Acupuncture Treatment
明堂孔穴针灸治要

My Understanding of Bian Que
扁鹊心书

New Book on Child Care
幼幼新书

New Illustrated Manual on the Points for Acupuncture and Moxibustion on the Bronze Figure
新铸铜人腧穴针灸图经

Old History of the Tang Dynasty
旧唐书

Orthodox Manual of Surgery
外科正宗

Outlaws of the Marsh
水浒传

Plain Questions
素问

Precious Book for Prescriptions
卫济宝书

Prescriptions for Traumatology
伤科方书

Prescriptions for Treating the Heart
医心方

Records of the Historian
史记

Reference for the Eight Extraordinary Channels
奇经八脉考

Renzhai Guide to Diagnosis and Prescriptions
仁斋直指附遗方论

Revised Canon of Herbs
新修本草

Rites of Zhou
周礼

Secret Prescriptions for the Treatment of Fracture and Reunion
理伤续断秘方

Secret Prescriptions Revealed by a Provincial Governor
外台秘要

Shen Nong's Canon of Herbs
神农本草经

Source of Diseases, The
诸病源候论

Standard Treatments in Diseases
证治准绳

Supplementary Golden Prescriptions
千金翼方

Supplement to Materia Medica
本草纲目拾遗

Surgery Cases
外科理例

Treatise on Febrile and Other Diseases
伤寒杂病论

Treatise on Febrile Diseases
伤寒论

Vital Pivot
灵枢

Yellow Emperor's Canon of Medicine, The
黄帝内经

Zhuang Zi
庄子

Zuoqiu Ming's Enlargement of the Spring and Autumn Annals
春秋左传

CHRONOLOGICAL TABLE OF CHINESE DYNASTIES

Xia	c. 21st-16th century B.C.
Shang	c. early 16th-11th century B.C.
Western Zhou	c. 11th century-770 B.C.
Eastern Zhou	770-221 B.C.
Spring and Autumn Period	770-476 B.C.
Warring States Period	475-221 B.C.
Qin	221-207 B.C.
Western Han	206 B.C.-A.D. 24
Eastern Han	25-220
Three Kingdoms	220-280
Western Jin	265-316
Eastern Jin	317-420
Southern and Northern Dynasties	420-589
Sui	581-618
Tang	618-907
Five Dynasties	907-979
Song	960-1279
Liao	916-1125
Kin	1115-1234
Yuan	1271-1368
Ming	1368-1644
Qing	1644-1911

ABOUT THE AUTHOR

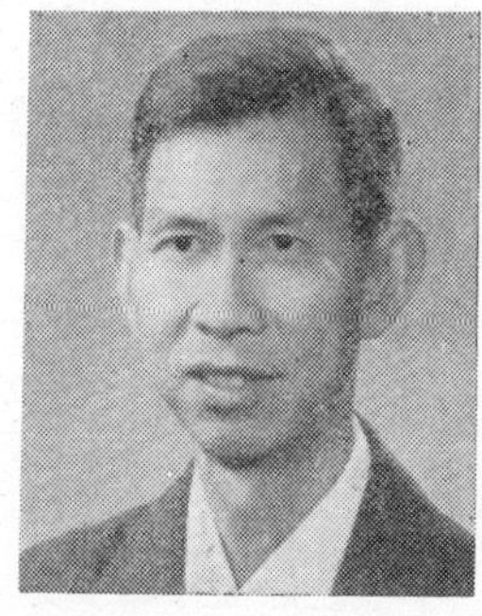

Fu Weikang, born in 1930 in China's Fujian Province, graduated in 1957 from the Shanghai First Medical College. He is now an associate professor and the Curator of the Museum of Medicine at the Shanghai College of Traditional Chinese Medicine, where he has been working since 1959, and Director of the college's Teaching and Research Section of the History of Chinese Medicine.

He was elected to the standing committee of the Society of the History of Chinese Medicine in 1979, and also serves as a council member of the Society of the History of Chinese Science and Technology, the Association of China's Museums of Natural Science and the Chinese Anthropological Society.

His publications include *The History of Chinese Acupuncture and Moxibustion* and *Lecture Notes of the History of Chinese Medicine.*